Delaying the Onset of Late-Life Dysfunction

Robert N. Butler, MD, is the Chairman and Brookdale Professor of the Henry L. Schwartz Department of Geriatrics and Adult Development at the Mount Sinai Medical Center, the first department of geriatrics in a U.S. medical school. From 1975 to 1982 he was the first director of the National Institute on Aging of the National Institutes of Health. In 1990, he cofounded the International Leadership Center on Longevity and Society, which studies the impact of longevity upon society and its institutions. In 1976, Dr. Butler won the Pulitzer prize for his book, *Why Survive? Being Old in America.* He is co-author of the books, *Aging and Mental Health* and *Love and Sex After 60.*

Jacob A. Brody, MD, is an internationally renowned expert in the epidemiology of health and disease in aging populations. From 1977 to l985, he was Associate Director of the National Institute on Aging and founded their epidemiology program. From 1985 to 1992, he served as Dean of the School of Public Health at the Health Sciences Center, University of Illinois in Chicago, where he is now Professor of Epidemiology and Professor of Research Medicine. Dr. Brody is the author and co-author of over 200 publications including studies of human brucellosis in Alaska, Parkinsonism-dementia in Guam, vesicular stomatitis virus in Panama, estrogen-replacement therapy, as well as trends and projections concerning the health of the elderly in the U.S. and the role of schools of public health in modern society.

Delaying the Onset of Late-Life Dysfunction

Robert N. Butler, MD

Jacob A. Brody, MD

Editors

 Springer Publishing Company

Springer Publishing Company, Inc.
536 Broadway
New York, NY 10012-3955

Cover design: *Tom Yabut*
Production Editor: *Joyce Noulas*
Associate Editor: *Kathryn R. Gertz*

95 96 97 98 99 / 5 4 3 2 1

Library of Congress Cataloging-in-Publication Data

Delaying the onset of late-life dysfuntion / Robert N. Butler, Jacob
A. Brody, editors.
      p. cm.
   Includes bibliographical references and index.
   ISBN 0-8261-8880-X
   1. Longevity. 2. Aging. 3. Chronic diseases—Prevention
4. Medicine, Preventive. I. Butler, Robert N., 1927–
II. Brody, Jacob A., 1931–
   [DNLM: 1. Aging. 2. Aged. 3. Chronic Disease—in old age.
   4. Primary Prevention—in old age. 5. Health promotion. 6. Quality
of Life. WT 104 D343 1995]
   QP85.D35   1995
613'.0438—dc20
DNLM/DLC
for Library of Congress   94-23931

Printed in the United States of America

Contents

Contributors

John Allman, PhD
California Institute of
  Technology–Division of
  Biology
Pasadena, CA 91125

Piero Anversa, MD
Department of Medicine
New York Medical College
Valhalla, NY 10595

Carl W. Cotman, PhD
Department of Psychobiology
University of
  California–Irvine
Irvine, CA 92717

Debra J. Decker, PhD
Scripps Clinic and Research
  Foundation
University of California at
  San Diego
La Jolla, CA 92037

William J. Evans, PhD
Director, Noll Laboratory for
  Human Performance
  Research
The Pennsylvania State
  University
University Park, PA 16802

Caleb E. Finch, PhD
Andrus Gerontology Center
University of Southern
  California
Los Angeles, CA 90089

Jon W. Gordon, MD, PhD
Department of OB/GYN
The Mount Sinai Medical
  Center
New York, NY 10029

Nikki J. Holbrook, PhD
Gene Expression in Aging
  Section
National Institute on Aging
Baltimore, MD 21224

Norman R. Klinman, MD
Scripps Clinic and Research
    Foundation
University of California at
    San Diego
La Jolla, CA 92037

Thierry H. Lejemtel, MD
Department of Cardiology
Albert Einstein College of
    Medicine
Bronx, NY 10461

Phyllis-Jean Linton, PhD
San Diego Regional Cancer
    Center
San Diego, CA 92121

Robert M. Sapolsky, PhD
Department of Biological
    Sciences
Stanford University
Stanford, CA 94305

Edmund H. Sonnenblick, MD
Albert Einstein College of
    Medicine
Bronx, New York 10461

Acknowledgments

The Brookdale Foundation has been a major supporter of the Henry L. Schwartz Department of Geriatrics and Adult Development at Mount Sinai Medical Center since the Department's inception in 1982. Once again, we would like to extend our heartfelt thanks to the Brookdale Foundation Group for providing support for "Strategies to Delay Dysfunction in Later Life," a symposium commemorating the 10th anniversary of the Department of Geriatrics and Adult Development, and the preparation of this book, which is based on that symposium.

We would like to extend special thanks to Merck & Company, the National Institute on Aging, the National Institute of Arthritis and Musculoskeletal and Skin Disease, the National Institute of Deafness and Other Communication Disorders, and the Alliance for Aging Research, for additional financial support.

The following organizations also contributed support that was much appreciated: The Jewish Home and Hospital for Aged, the American Association of Homes for the Aged, the American Association of Retired Persons, Marion Merrell Dow, Sandoz Pharmaceuticals Corporation, the UpJohn Company, and Wyeth Ayerest Laboratories.

Finally, we would like to thank Kathryn Gertz for all her diligent help in preparing this manuscript.

This symposium was the first in a series of symposia sponsored by the International Longevity Center (U.S.).

Introduction: Revolution in Longevity 1

Robert N. Butler

In the late 1700's, the average life expectancy at birth was 35 years. At the turn of the 20th century, it was 47 years on average, and only 3% of the population made it past age 65. The 20th century revolution in longevity has led to an added 25 or more years of life. In the U.S. today, average life expectancy at birth has jumped to 75, and a full 80% of all deaths occur after age 65. In addition, people over 85 now constitute the fastest growing segment of our population. Unfortunately, though, health maintenance among the elderly has not quite kept pace. While it is true that we have postponed death, we have not yet been able to delay the age of onset of a variety of distressing disorders associated with growing older. Dementia, arthritis, diminished hearing and visual acuity, incontinence, hip fracture—all continue to occur at the same age as they did in the past. The chronic, non-fatal disorders of longevity destroy the quality of life and sap society's resources.

Does this mean that longer life necessarily brings with it more years of chronic disability? The latest evidence seems to support the concept that it does *not* and that we can indeed defer disease and dysfunction. Such postponement can become the most effective means of prevention, and prevention is essential if we are to reduce the staggering social and economic costs of disease. The papers collected in this volume suggest scientific strategies and areas of research that could eventually lead to successful prevention of the diseases and disabilities of old age.

Were it possible to postpone physical dependency among persons 65 and above in the aggregate, it is estimated that $5 billion or more per month in public and private spending could be saved.* This does not represent a one-time saving only, but would establish a new lower basis for further expenditures in the future, assuming other variables remain constant. Such deferral is complex, and we need to understand better all the actual and biomedical implications, since *all* variables are not likely to remain the same. As a result of deferral, for example, either increased robustness or frailty could occur, new useful medical findings could be introduced in the meantime, cures for diseases found, and so on.

There are basically two ways of increasing longevity. One is through health promotion and disease prevention. The other is through basic research involving all the rich new possibilities of molecular and cellular biology and applying the results. Increasingly, these two methods will be combined. For example, if we are able to identify a gene for a specific disease such as colon cancer, an individual with such a marker could have the opportunity to alter his or her behavior accordingly, eating less fat and having more frequent check-ups, for example.

We need not, however—indeed, we *should* not—wait for the future findings of biology to apply what we already know. This becomes evident when we consider the status of health behavior in the United States today. Exercise, particularly aerobic activity and resistance training, has been shown through outstanding clinical investigations to reduce physical frailty, and yet 71% of people do not exercise. Pneumonia and its complications are among the top ten causes of death, and yet 86% of people over age 65 do not receive the pneumococ-

*Data from the Alliance for Aging Research, which used Health Care Financing Administration data to calculate the savings from delaying the onset of disability in terms of hospital and doctor costs ($1.8 billion per month); nursing home costs ($3.2 billion per month); and home care costs ($.3 billion per month); total savings = $5.3 billion per month.

cal vaccine. Some 10,000 people die of the flu in an epidemic and 70,000 succumb when there is a major epidemic. Yet 50% of persons 65 and over do not get their autumn flu shot. Lung cancer attributable to tobacco use has surpassed breast cancer among women, and yet nearly 30% of Americans still smoke. In fact, by all accounts, tobacco and alcohol are directly responsible for the top two causes of premature death—heart disease and cancer. Even so, there are 18 million Americans with alcohol problems, 10 million of whom are considered to have hard-core alcoholic disorders. In addition, the vast majority of Americans continue to eat high fat diets even though such foods have been shown to dramatically increase the risk of heart disease and cancer.

Health promotion and disease prevention are a dual responsibility that must be shared by the individual and society. The individual needs to adopt a lower risk lifestyle and society must educate the public, support biomedical research, and elect government officials who will introduce legislation to maintain and improve public health. An example of this synergy is the issue of smoking and the necessary avoidance of active and passive smoke. There is no question that we need to continue various efforts to help current American smokers quit the habit. However, since 1964, when the Surgeon General's report on smoking was issued, there has been progress, including a steady decrease in the number of Americans who smoke and more protection of nonsmokers through legislation requiring smoke-free environments. It is possible that the present debate over the addictiveness of nicotine could lead to even greater restrictions on tobacco. This is an example of what can happen when individuals and society collaborate to prevent disease.

It is *never* too late to introduce new health habits. Indeed, the economic consequences of *not* doing so, and consequently of not preventing or postponing dysfunction, are staggering. Inaction is fatal and costly. We can see that now as we continue to pay for the care of people with disease rather than paying to prevent disease. The economic cost of disease to our society is enormous in terms of both direct cost—i.e., resources spent on hospitals, physicians, labs, pharmacies, other goods and services that go along with medical care — and indirect costs, meaning not only loss of productivity by the patient but also by the members of that individual's family and other unpaid caregivers.

Where, then, would our health dollars best be spent? To begin with, public dissemination of information is absolutely essential if people are to make informed choices. Federal and state efforts in that direction have improved in recent years. Dr. Julius Richmond, who became Surgeon General in 1976, led the way in advancing health promotion and disease prevention. Human behavior can change and such change can be maintained. Indeed, informed choices lead to lifestyle changes which, in turn, lead to major beneficial transformations in health and social well-being.

We know, too, that economic determinants change behavior. Tobacco and alcohol taxes actually reduce consumption, especially among the young. In Canada, for example, hefty taxes on cigarettes have had a quantitative impact on tobacco use. How useful it would be if there were an even greater investment in social and behavioral research to help us understand better other incentives and disincentives to lifestyle change. It is especially important to disentangle the roles of genes and socialization involved in addictive behavior. Clinical studies can help us understand many physiological and pathophysiological issues and can lead us to solutions which will delay or prevent disability, such as the studies discussed by William Evans, one of our contributors, on the loss of lean muscle mass and the beneficial effects of exercise in even the very old. Another example is the currently ongoing Progesterone Estrogen Preventive Intervention (PEPI) trial at the National Institutes of Health (NIH) which will shed new light on the increased vulnerability to heart disease and osteoporosis experienced by post-menopausal women and the efficacy and safety of hormone replacement therapy. Most of all, we must invest in basic biology, especially the "new biology"—recombinant DNA, hybridoma, and transgenic technologies—which is the wave of the future in both prevention and treatment.

Mega-science projects such as the Human Genome Project, which may lead to numerous contributions to human health, should be cooperative, multi-national efforts. Animal models remain critical to scientific success as well. Animal resources, especially aging animals, are both essential and expensive.

Among the basic biological questions: What is a symptomatic or phenotypic threshold of a disease? How many cells do we need to lose in the macula before visual impairment occurs? Or in the substantia nigra before Parkinson's disease develops? What do we do about infectious disease and the fact that microbes have become so skilled at survival? As Joshua Lederberg and colleagues (1992) described so well in the volume *Emerging Infections* commissioned by the Institute of Medicine. And what about certain cancers that may have been predetermined genetically years before but may reveal themselves only after certain changes in the environment or in relation to the passage of time? How might we forestall cancer? How do we maintain the immune system? Study of the mechanism of metastases should be a fruitful field. The expression of genetic disease, the ecology of disease in general, is another area of vast importance.

The ultimate goal of this trend of thought, of course, is a disease-free old age in which people remain healthy and functional until the end. It is the classic dream of gerontologists illustrated so eloquently by the 19th-century poem "The Deacon's Masterpiece or The Wonderful One-Hoss Shay," written by the great doctor and poet Oliver Wendell Holmes (1955). In effect, we could postpone all disease until a predetermined length of life is over so that we could "go to pieces," as Holmes put it, "All at once, and nothing first,—/Just as bubbles do when they burst." The goal is to counter the famous Gompertzian formulation, which states that the force of mortality proceeds exponentially with age (especially after age 30), doubling every 7 years, to change the pace of overall aging or the aging processes of specific organs or bodily systems, and ultimately to reset the biological clock. Delaying dysfunction means reducing both the length and the amount of dependency. If we carry this bold concept through to its ultimate conclusion, all disease and disability would be postponed literally beyond death, the very point at which the biological clock has run out!

What are other mechanisms of delay? The redundancy of systems in the body and its surprising plasticity or ability to repair itself are parts of the biological basis for the mechanism of delay. Caloric restriction, first studied in depth by Clive McCay, causes delay of dysfunction and even of death. Control of free radical damage is relevant and gene regulation is key. Moderation of stress may restrain brain aging, as our contributor Robert Sapolsky points out. Delaying immunosenescence may prove to be a powerful weapon against disability, as may growth factors. In general, gene therapy approaches seem the most dramatic.

How much should we invest in such biomedical research? Indeed, in all of science? Should it be at the rate of GNP or greater than the GNP rate? As Nobel economist Robert Solow demonstrated, science constitutes a considerable contribution to the economic progress of our country. Should we invest a percentage of health care expenditures in medical research? Yes, a sizable percentage! Today, on average, less than 20% of approved grants are funded by the NIH. Congress and the Executive Branch of government should double the base of support to 40%. (When Eisenhower was President, all approved grants were funded.) Certainly there is a great cost to doing nothing. In the case of Alzheimer's disease, for example, it has been projected that by the year 2040, as the number of older people increases, the number of Alzheimer's patients will grow to three to five times the current count, which means that we could be facing a $300 billion to $500 billion national expenditure for Alzheimer's disease alone.

Aging research is worth doing, especially in the context of a onger life expectancy since we want to keep cutting disability rates while lengthening life. Thus far, indications are that we are on the right track. American physician James Fries (1980) predicted the "compression of morbidity," which, he asserted optimistically, would occur following successful health promotion, disease prevention, and research. Recent reports by Manton, Corder, and Stallard (1993) suggest that disability rates have indeed declined, both *manifest* disability as a consequence of medical responses, assistive devices and housing improvements, and *inherent* disability rates.

The human desire is *not* to take longer to die but to live longer in good health through deferral of non-fatal as well as fatal conditions. This is an important strategy for biomedical science policy to support. From that perspective, biomedical research is the ultimate method of prevention, the ultimate service to humankind, and the ultimate cost containment strategy.

But can we really plan research, or can we only provide the resources and sketch general priorities? On the one hand, scientists want money to do their work and freedom to explore as they wish. On the other hand, the public—which provides the tax dollars—has a vested interest in the way in which these funds are expended. Taxpayers ultimately finance science and technology, and they want results.

How can we match these simple desires: to have scientific freedom as well as reasonable and productive planning? Perhaps the common ground is the provision of basic resources and the assurance that funds channeled into mega-science projects will not subtract funds from investigator-initiated research. We should sponsor major initiatives to tackle specific problems but avoid micro-management. Science as a profession is not only a matter of luck. Furthermore, it is troubling that in these austere times, review groups have become very conservative and do not support risky research proposals. There should, however, always be a set-aside for high-risk scientific studies.

I believe that our nation must strengthen its support of basic science and preserve individual investigator-initiated research. It has been demonstrated over and over again that undifferentiated, untargeted science is the basis of extraordinary discoveries that meet human needs. Thus we are always engaged in an effort to, on the one hand, balance the public's expectations—reflected in what I call the "health politics of anguish" and advocacy within our democratic form of government—and, on the other hand, the need to preserve scientific freedom and the possibility of serendipity. Flexible planning involving priority setting and planning of resources is demonstrated in the National Academy of Science/Institute of Medicine's *Extending Life, Enhancing Life* (Lonergan, 1991) the most recent national research plan on aging. It is also important for biomedical science policy to be compatible with the eagerly awaited national health reforms. For example, with the expected emphasis on primary care and prevention, it would be most regrettable if current health reforms led to stifling or undue control of science and technology.

Increasing attention has been paid in the 20th century to the role of genes and the environment, broadly defined to include lifestyle and the quality of our air and water. Not until the past 20 years, though, has significant attention been focused upon the role of aging of the organism. Yet aging brings about increased vulnerability to disease and disability, and it is necessary to understand all antecedents of dysfunction. The 21st century is likely to bring an even greater expansion of research interest in all three interconnected antecedents to disease: genetics, the environment, and aging—for the purpose of postponement as well as cure. The challenge is to delay dysfunction at a rate that outpaces the increase in life expectancy.

REFERENCES

Fries, J.F. (1980). Aging, natural death, and the compression of morbidity. *New England Journal of Medicine* 303:130–125.

Holmes, O.W. (1955). The deacon's masterpeice or, the wonderful "one-hoss shay." In Oscar Williams (ed.), *American Verse from Colonial Days to the Present.* New York: Pocket Books.

Lederberg, J. (1992). *Emerging infections: Microbal threats to health in the U.S.* Washington, D.C.: National Academy Press.

Lonergan, E.T. (Ed.). (1991). Extending life, enhancing life. A national research agenda on aging. Washington, D.C.: National Academy Press.

Manton, K.G., Corder, L.S., & Stallard, E. (1993). Estimates of change in chronic disability and institutional incidence and prevalence rates in the U.S. elderly population from 1982, 1984, and 1989 National Long-Term Care Survey. *Journal of Gerontology: Social Sciences*, vol. 48, no. 4, S153–S166.

Postponement As Prevention In Aging

2

Jacob A. Brody

INTRODUCTION

This chapter begins with two assertions and an illustration, and the remainder is devoted to the history and development of the concept of postponement as prevention. The first assertion is the observation that the human body is so well made that it easily outlives its joints, its cognitive and memory capacities, its vision, its hearing its sphincters and numerous other functions. The second is that efforts directed at the precursors of disability are the most promising and potentially effective mechanisms available to prevent chronic diseases and attendant dysfunction (Brody, 1987).

The potential power of postponement is illustrated in Figure 2.1. Hip fracture rates in American females rise suddenly at about age 40, and thereafter increase exponentially, doubling each 5 to 6 years. (Brody, Farmer, & White, 1984; Farmer, White, Brody, & Bailey, 1984; Kellie & Brody, 1990). If we could delay the sudden rise by 6 years, the exponential portion of the curve would have one less doubling and hence we half the number of hip fractures. Hip fracture is closely related to osteoporosis and progressive bone degeneration. We are already practicing various strategies to delay osteoporosis and hip fracture. These include behavioral modifications such as diet and exercise, thera-

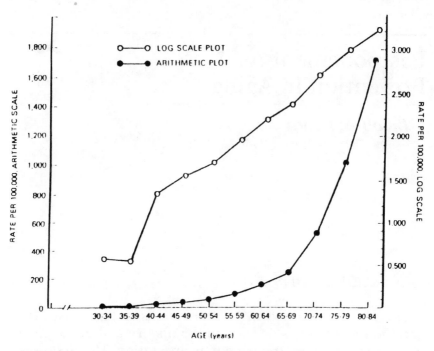

FIGURE 2.1 Age-specific hip fracture incidence among United States white women. (*Source*: National Hospital Discharge Survey, National Center for Health Statistics.)

peutic regimens using hormones, medication and vitamins and finally, taking precautions to avoid falls in older people. A more powerful approach is through research focusing on bone degeneration and determining specific factors regulating osteoblasts, osteoclasts, calcium utilization and excretion etc., in order to find mechanisms which slow down what we now accept as a normal pattern of bone loss with age.

POPULATION SHIFTS IN THE 20TH CENTURY AND THEIR IMPLICATIONS

In 1991 there were 2,165,000 deaths in the United States, of which 484,000 or 22% occurred in women 80 years of age and over (Annual Summary of Births, Marriages, Divorces, and Deaths, 1991). At the same time, specific mortality rates for women age 80 and over is at an all time low. Longevity in the 20th century has increased at an astounding rate. It is not an overstatement to point out that our social and medical efforts are struggling to catch up with the new realities. In 1900 only a quarter of the population survived to age 65 (U.S. Dept. of Health and Human Services, 1991), while in 1990 73% achieved this age, with half of those deaths occurring after age 80.

The pattern of reduction in mortality this century, however, has not been smooth over time or easily explainable. In Figure 2.2A we note the mortality rate per 100,000 for all ages fell from 1,720 to 861 between 1900 and 1990. Almost half of this remarkable decrease was completed by 1920. It is doubtful that the hand of the physician or the social planner was prominent in the period during which the greatest mortality reduction occurred. Instead, it appears that improved living environments, nutrition, and better sanitation were the major factors in the decline.

Among those 65 and over, mortality had declined barely 5% by 1920 (Fig. 2.2B) indicating that the older population was less affected by the factors that had caused the remarkable change in the general population. Those 65 and over, however, caught up by about 1950 when one half of the decline in mortality for that age group was completed. The era between 1920 and 1950 was an eventful one in American history, with such notable occurrences as World War II, The Great Depression, the beginning of Social Security, and Prohibition. While one might speculate on which of these and other events caused the decline in mortality by mid-century, factors related to specific social or medical interventions are not likely to have been major contributors. From 1950 to 1970, the overall mortality rate was generally unchanged with an actual increase in mortality for those age 65 and over (Fig. 2.2B). This apparent quiescence reassured policy makers and planners and in a sense lulled them into a false assumptions of stable predict-

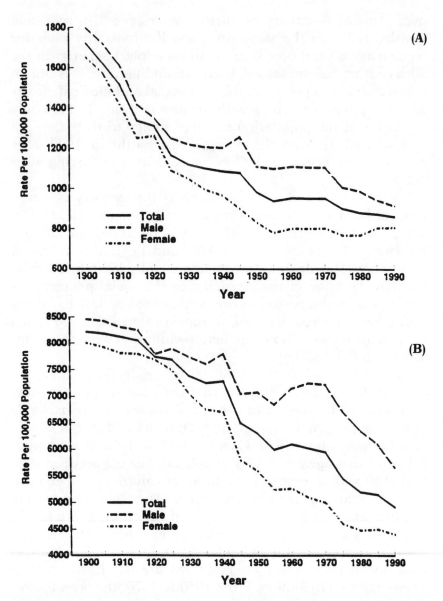

FIGURE 2.2 Mortality rates for years 1900–1990, by gender. (A) All ages. (B) Ages 65 and over. (*Source*: National Center for Health Statistics (U.S. Public Health Service), various volumes of "Vital Statistics of the United States.")

ability (U.S. National Center for Health Statistics, 1964) as life expectancy approached the biblical three score and ten.

Since about 1968 mortality rates have followed a persistent decline. The rates, however, are much greater for the population 65 and over than for the general population (Fig. 2.2B), which has resulted in a disproportionate accumulation of the oldest and most vulnerable sector of our population. Can this recent trend be credited to medical and social interventions? Certainly some benefits accrue, perhaps the most powerful being reduction of blood pressure and the improvement of medical care through Medicare and other health insurance programs (U.S. National Center for Health Statistics, 1983). Social, medical, and public health efforts have included reduction in smoking and the promotion of improvements in lifestyle through diet and exercise. While some scientific documentation of the benefits of diet and exercise exists, the quantifiable gains are small (Paffenberger et al., 1993). Careful analysis of the data on powerful promoters of human health and longevity such as not smoking and the use of antihypertensive agents reveals that for neither of these parameters had success been sufficient or timely enough to explain the decline of mortality in the elderly in 1968 (Stallones, 1982). The major impact of blood pressure control and reduced smoking is yet to be fully realized and thus we are likely to experience even greater gains in longevity in future years.

The most remarkable change in mortality patterns for adults in the 20th century occurred for ischemic heart disease which started to decline in about 1968. As is true of many great medical triumphs, though, the results are not easily attributed to our own constructive action (Ewbank & Wray, 1980). Tuberculosis, for example, was the number one killer in the United States at the turn of the century even though TB mortality had been declining since 1856 and despite the fact that the tuberculosis bacillus was not identified until 1882 and specific therapies were only introduced in the late 1940s. Scarlet fever is another case in point. Between 1870 and 1900 there was a precipitous decline in deaths from this disease and yet sulfa-drugs and penicillin were not in common use until World War II and after. Nor are shifts confined to infectious diseases. Mortality from accidents among the elderly has been declining rapidly since 1950 (Brody, 1987), and conversion hysteria, one of Freud's most frequent diagnoses seems to have vanished. Mortality from stomach cancer and stroke has been declining since at least 1950 in the United States and perhaps for longer (Brock & Brody, 1984). The rapid decline in mortality from ischemic heart disease and attendant acute myocardial infarction occurred in the late 1960s, but as mentioned, the extent to which this was the result of our own medical and social interventions is certainly questioned as is the sense of control of our survival which this phenomenon generated (Brody, 1987).

It appears that acute myocardial infarction is a 20th century disease and disaster. There is no mention in the literature of the classical heart attack before 1900. The generally accepted first medical reference is in 1912 by Herrick (1982). It is possible that the medical profession simply had failed to observe or define heart attacks and separate them from acute gastrointestinal or pulmonary disease. A heart attack is, however, a notable event with crushing chest pain, and pain radiating down the left arm, syncope and sweating. Even if physicians missed the diagnosis, surely authors and playwrights who eloquently describe medical events should have written about something as dramatic as a myocardial infarction. There are, however, no good descriptions of heart attacks in a literature which abounds in detailed passages about gout, apoplexy, epilepsy, cancer, tuberculosis, etc.

I suggest that while the occasional case of acute myocardial infraction occurred prior to 1900, the event was rare. At the turn of the century, though, a set of circumstances emerged which created the conditions necessary for the disease to become noticed and increasingly dominant. Among these events were the introduction of cigarette smoking, a shift in diet and particularly fat ingestion, and a more urban and less physically strenuous work and lifestyle. The stage was set and the eruption occurred.

Mortality from heart attacks has been declining in the United States since 1968, but this decrease was not observed throughout the world and notably not in such countries as Sweden (Welin, Larsson, Svardsudd, Wilhelmsen, & Tibblin, 1981) and Japan (Kimura, 1983), where life expectancy is greater than in the United States. The scenario I suggest is that acute myocardial infarction was introduced and flourished at a time in which most causes of death were receding. When acute and infectious disease dwindled early in the century, the dominant killer became heart disease and still is.

About half of all deaths are caused by some form of heart disease of which a large fraction is the result of acute myocardial infarction. As Figure 2.2 shows, there was steady decline in overall mortality through World War II. At that point, mortality reached a plateau and even rose a bit. It is likely that during the 1950s and 1960s the primary forces which had reduced mortality during the early part of the century were slowing down while mortality from acute myocardial infarction was rising. The rapid decline in deaths from acute myocardial infarction commenced in the late 1960s at a time when only modest changes in smoking patterns, exercise, and diet had occurred. The entire epidemic affected men far more than women, and it seems that rather small changes in risk factors were sufficient to cause an abrupt decline in outcome. Thus the 20th century saw the rise and fall of deaths from acute myocardial infarctions. Age specific mortality rates in the United States would have shown a general persistent and much smoother decline for the entire century had it not been for the remarkable appearance of mortality from acute myocardial infarction (Brody, 1985).

Given this insight, the driving force in the extension of life expectancy appears more closely to fit a pattern of the release of something intrinsic in humans rather than a decline in cause-specific mortality. For at least the past century we have been moving nearer to our genetic potential. There is an analogy and almost surely a relationship between increasing survival and the consistent observation that for more than a century people have been getting taller with successive generations. The factors likely to have lead to the extension of growth are the reduction of frequent and severe infections and better nutrition in the early formative years. There is evidence in some populations that growth may have reached a plateau either temporarily or perhaps permanently (Abraham, Johnson, & Najjars, 1977). We postulated (Brody, 1985, 1987) that we are observing people better equipped for survival, since with each successive generation the cohort of children more closely approaches the maximum human growth potential. This phenomenon sets up cohorts with successively improved trajectories for survival. Indeed, it is not accidental that current longevity was preceded by increased growth in childhood.

OBSERVATIONS IN A LONGER LIVING SPECIES

The tumbling up in populations of long-living people was alluded to above and will be expanded upon in this section. Several hypotheses and concepts emerge because of the ability to make observations on 8th, 9th, and 10th decades of life. Many diseases, conditions, and social situations are associated with aging. We have been trying to sort out two distinct types of associations which occur (Brody, 1990; Brody & Schneider, 1986). Words can be arbitrary, but for convenience of presentation I had been using two terms: *age-dependent* versus *age-related* diseases and conditions, the former being diseases which increase the longer we live and the latter being diseases which occur at a defined age and then cease to occur or diminish. Recently (Finch, 1990; Carey, Liedo, Orozco, & Vaupel, 1992) two colleagues whose native languages are not English suggested more precise and accurate terminology which I shall use in this manuscript. "Age-dependent" will become *aging-dependent*, and "age-related" will become *age-dependent*.

Aging-dependent diseases are those which rise steadily with age, accumulating as we live longer. These diseases follow the basic Gompertz logarithmic curve of mortality in which

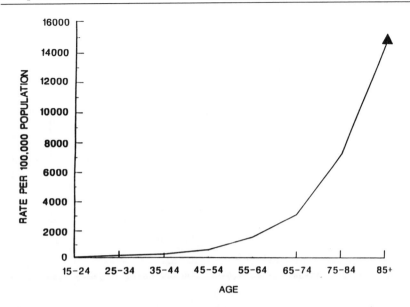

FIGURE 2.3 Mortality rates for selected causes by age group, 1988. (*Source*: Vital Statistics of the United States, Volume 11–Mortality, Part A, 1988. National Center for Health Statistics.)

deaths from all causes rise exponentially from about age 35 (Fig. 2.3). The Gompertz curve seems to hold up well over many years of study and in numerous species, although deviations have been observed (Guralnik, LaCroix, Everett, & Kovar, 1989; Dunn, Rudberg, Furner, & Cassel, 1992). Figure 2.4 presents mortality from heart disease—the major age-dependent disease—superimposed on the basic mortality curve shown above. These curves have similar patterns since half of all deaths are from heart disease. A large array of other *aging-dependent* diseases and conditions include cerebrovascular disease, dementias, vision and hearing loss, type II diabetes and altered glucose metabolism, hip fracture, osteoporosis, Parkinson's disease, specific infections such as pneumococcal pneumonia (actually exceeds the Gompertz curve), constipation, incontinence, signs of depression, social isolation and living alone, widowhood, and institutionalization.

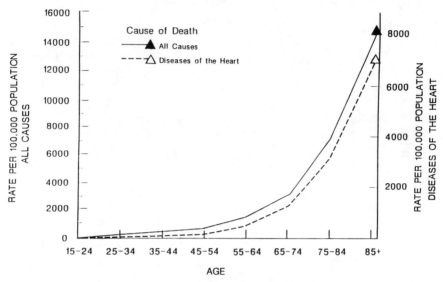

FIGURE 2.4 Mortality rates for selected causes by age group, 1988. (*Source*: Vital Statistics of the United States, Volume 11–Mortality, Part A, 1988.)

While it is tempting to consider aging itself as a disease which is *aging-dependent*, this is not a helpful approach. It is more useful to consider aging as a series of risk factors providing fertile soil for numerous events. In other words, the accumulation of normal aging characteristics creates a threshold beyond which there is increased susceptibility for an array of outcomes. This language avoids a discussion of normal aging and implies that there is no use or reality for the term natural death.

With age and perhaps at a rate even steeper than the Gompertz curve comes the occurrence of more than one *aging-dependent* disease or condition. These are now commonly called co-morbidities and presentations; methodologies for studying these detrimental fellow travelers are increasingly available (Guralnik et al., 1989; Dunn et al., 1992).

The second class of diseases and conditions associated with age we termed *age-dependent* (Brody & Schneider, 1986). *Age-*

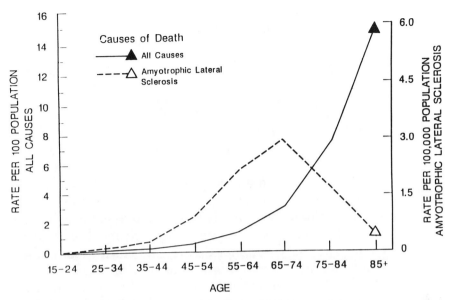

FIGURE 2.5 Mortality rates for all causes by age group, 1988. (*Source*: Vital Statistics of the United States, Volume 11–Mortality, Part A, 1988. National Center for Health Statistics.)

dependent diseases occur at a certain time in life and if one passes through the susceptible period, the disease is much less likely to develop. The prototype of an *age-dependent* disease is amyotrophic lateral sclerosis (Fig. 2.5) in which deaths do not occur before age 40 or 45 and rarely after age 70. Multiple sclerosis is another *age-dependent* disease; onset occurs in the mid to late teens and deaths decline beyond age 50. In fact, a surprising number of diseases and conditions are *age-depen-dent*. Schizophrenia is generally confined to late adolescence and early adulthood. New cases of peptic ulcer rarely occur after age 45. Gout does not appear for the first time beyond age 50 and nor does ulcerative colitis. Hemorrhoids occur in middle-age and alcoholism declines rapidly after age 50.

Also *age-dependent* are slow viruses which by definition produce diseases in which there is no immune component. In laboratory animals the incubation period between inoculation and disease is fixed in duration regardless of age. Therefore, it is difficult to understand why slow virus diseases in humans do not increase with age as occurs in *aging-dependent* disease. The most important slow virus diseases—Kuru, Jakob-Creutzfeldt disease, subacute sclerosis panencephalitis, and the Gerstmann-Straussler syndrome—occur in younger people while primary multifocal leukoencephalopathy occurs in late middle life and with AIDS.

Cancers appear to be on the cusp of our hypothesis. Mortality from all cancers and cardiovascular disease is shown in Figure 2.6. Cancer rises in a linear fashion from about age 40 to 75 and then mortality seems to plateau. There are now some data in countries which have had enough experience in the 9th and 10th decades to suggest that age-specific cancer mortality may actually decline. Clearly, mortality from cancer does not increase exponentially and it is probably useful to consider it an *age-dependent* condition. This is of particular relevance since animal studies reveal that mutagenesis increases in an exponential manner with age. Although mutagenesis occurs, the energy to propel the process into a full blown cancer seems to wane perhaps with the waning of many immune functions and other forms of host inertia. At age 65 to 69, 30% of all deaths are from cancer, while for deaths in those 85 and over only 10% are caused by cancer.

The theme of this symposium is strategies to delay dysfunction. For *aging-dependent* diseases we expand on the possibilities of postponement of onset. Concerning *aging-dependent* diseases, though, the essential factor is to learn how to shepherd people through the critical age and by delaying onset we prevent the illness. There is no facile explanation for *age-dependent* conditions and why they cease to occur after a certain age. With infectious diseases it is usual to think of exhaustion of susceptibles preventing occurrence at later ages. With chronic disease we look for measurable genetic or environmental associations related to the pattern of occurrence or death to provide evidence that the available pool of patients has been exhausted. For most conditions, these patterns simply do not exist. It is likely that host alteration pre-

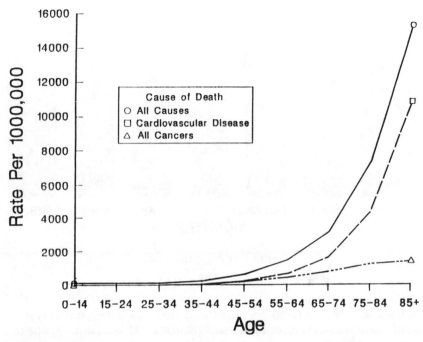

FIGURE 2.6 Mortality rates for selected causes by age group, 1988. (*Source*: Vital Statistics of the United States, Volume 11–Mortality, Part A, 1988. National Center for Health Statistics.)

vents some illnesses from occurring later in life. Examples could be hemorrhoids and gout or even the suggestion raised about cancer in which the body will no longer perform its role in pathogenesis. Exhaustion of susceptibles, however, would seem an unlikely explanation for most of these conditions or for the failure of occurrence in late life of peptic ulcer, glioblastoma, colitis, slow virus disease, or alcoholism.

MORTALITY, MORBIDITY AND THE POSTPONEMENT IMPERATIVE

To more adequately portray current and future mortality patterns we are developing a concept of Phase I and Phase II

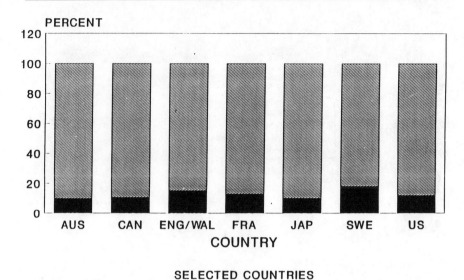

FIGURE 2.7   Proportion 65 years and over (as a percent of total population, selected countries). (*Source*: U.N. Demographic Yearbook, 1985.)

Mortality (Brody & Miles, 1990). Phase I Mortality is defined as the transitional period in the maturation of a population in which only 20% of deaths occur before age 65. Figure 2.7 illustrates that for most developed countries between 10 and 18% of the population is 65 and over, and in Figure 2.8 between 69 and 81% of all deaths in these countries occur at age 65 and over.

As expected there is a close relationship between the percent of the population age 65 and over and the percent of deaths in this age group (Fig. 2.9). Currently in Sweden about 18% are 65 and over, and 84% of all deaths occur in this population. Thus Sweden and many countries of Central and Northern Europe have already passed Phase I Mortality. In the United States in 1990, 12.5 to 13% of the population and 73% of deaths were in people 65 and over. Between the years 2005 and 2025 all developed countries will have approxi-

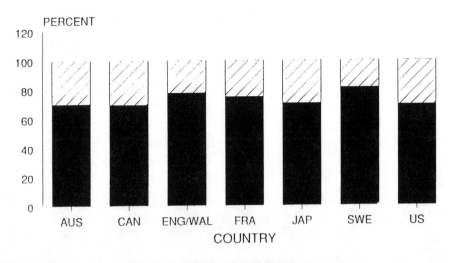

FIGURE 2.8 Proportion deaths 65 years and over (as percent of total deaths). (*Source*: U.N. Demographic Yearbook, 1985.)

mately 20% of their population 65 and over (Brody, Freels, & Miles, 1992). During the next century many of the developing countries will achieve this level (Kinsella, 1993; Miles &＊ Brody, in press).

Various data sources (Brody, 1987; Torrey, Kinsella, & Tauber, 1987; Olshansky, Carnes, & Cassel, 1993) suggest a steady state in developed countries after the year 2020, with about 20% of the population age 65 and over, which we define as Phase II Mortality. Approximately 15% of deaths would be occurring under age 65. With Phase II Mortality it would be appropriate to replace the use of percent of deaths to a rate analogous to the infant mortality rate and compare countries, regions, ethnic groups, and public health programs in relation to this new statistic (Brody & Miles, 1990).

In developed nations, between 70% and 80% of deaths in those 65 and over are from heart disease, stroke and cancer (Fig. 2.10). There are variations in this pattern from country

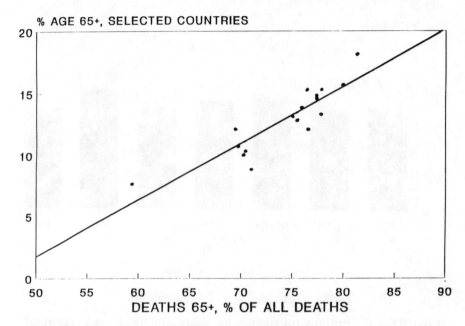

FIGURE 2.9 Population aged 65 years and over (percent total by percent deaths). (*Source*: U.N. Demographic Yearbook, 1986.)

to country and perhaps future health strategies will actually change the pattern. For the last 40 years, however, 70 to 80% of all deaths have been from these three causes (Sutherland, Persky, & Brody, 1990; Demographic Yearbook, 1986). Thus, the increase in life expectancy in the developed countries for almost the last half century results from the fact that these specific diseases produce death at later and later ages.

We are all aware that postponing death is a triumph, but there are reservations. Now that we are living longer, are we living better? For fatal diseases such as heart disease, cancer, and strokes are we living longer by lingering longer or has age of onset actually been postponed? There is no simple answer to this question and the sum of most studies suggests a modicum of postponement of onset and definitely more years of lingering.

An urgent area for study is the nonfatal *aging-dependent*

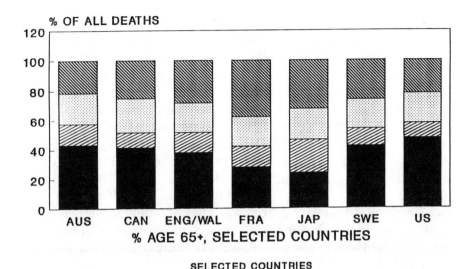

FIGURE 2.10 Selected causes of death, age 65+ percent heart, stroke, cancer, & other. (*Source*: U.N. Demographic Yearbook, 1986.)

diseases and conditions of aging. These diseases increase inexorably with age as discussed above and cause many of the conditions we fear most. With Phase I mortality upon us and Phase II only decades away, postponement is the main approach to prevention and delay in the population 65 and over. For this reason the discussion of hip fracture and postponement was presented at the beginning of this paper. Other nonfatal *aging-dependent* candidates for postponement include Alzheimer's disease and related dementias, loss of vision and hearing, arthritis, incontinence, and osteoporosis.

We have not directed enough serious attention to the concept of postponement and the enormous benefits to be accrued. Most of the fatal diseases and all of the nonfatal diseases we discussed increase exponentially with age. Postponing, therefore, has a magnified effect since delaying a process by one doubling will reduce by half the future incidence. We are living too long not to direct more of our efforts toward diseases which make aging a burdensome process.

For most nonfatal diseases we do not know at present if adding years to life expectancy this century has had any effect on the age at onset. Do we need glasses later in life? Has presbycusis been postponed? Is dementia or osteoarthritis occurring later in life? Adding 30 years to female life expectancy in the 1900s has had little or no impact on the age at menopause (Gosden, 1985). Disturbingly, the age-specific incidence of hip fracture has been rising during the last two decades (Bacon & Smith, in press; Boyce & Vesey, 1985; Brody, 1988; Zetterling, Elmerson, & Anderson, 1940–1983). Unless we know that increasing survival also postpones the age-specific onset of these non-fatal *aging-dependent* conditions, we are too lightly accepting that we will simply be living longer and sicker.

About 13 years ago Fries (1980) postulated optimistically that the limits of life expectancy were about 85 years and morbidity would be compressed and costs decline. While all would welcome this notion, many of us have faulted the solidity of the concept and the basic data and data assumptions (Brody, 1982; Crimmins, 1984; Meyers & Manton, 1984; Olshansky et al., 1990; Schneider & Brody, 1983). Indeed, in some populations life expectancy is already approaching Fries' 85 years. Recently, Manton and collaborators (Manton, Larry, & Stollard, in press; Manton, Stallard, & Tolley, 1991) published astounding increases in life expectancy in some population groups as well huge declines in age specific ADL and IADL scores of functional capacity in old, old populations. The techniques used require extensive modeling with many assumptions analogous to those which have earned economics the sobriquet of the dismal science. Manton does acknowledge that there will continue to be an absolute increase in costs because of population shifts. His data are obviously important and strain our credulity as biologists. David Hume wrote in *An Enquiry Concerning Human Understanding* that "no testimony is sufficient to establish a miracle, unless the testimony be of such a kind, that its falsehood would be more

miraculous than the fact which it endeavors to establish"
(1952). The essence of the scientific method is reproduceabil-
ity. Our Chicago group spearheaded by Olshansky and Furner
is attempting to do this before policy makers commit potentially serious errors.

CONCLUSIONS

We are living longer and more salubriously than ever. Science and society, however, are buffeted by projections of vast
further increases in longevity and at the same time bom-
barded by the gloom concerning long-term care, the costs of
health and the ever-augmenting disability and frailty of the
increasing aged population. It is important to reiterate that
we are mortal. Some increases in longevity will occur but
great leaps are unlikely and at present are patently unwel-
come since our social and medical institutions are not keeping up with the present reality.

As of yet, there is no evidence that we have delayed the onset of dementia, arthritis, diminished hearing and visual acuity, incontinence and hip fracture. These conditions are
closely related to normal aging. After a threshold of damaged
cellular or organ function, signs and symptoms emerge progressively. Their onset occurs in an exponential fashion typically doubling in incidence every 5 to 7 years. Postponement
of these diseases would have a tremendously beneficial impact on late life. Various mechanisms for postponing these
diseases are at hand. We know certain behaviors and medication will influence their appearance. We have not, however, re-
addressed our scientific thinking to the possibility that we
can slow down some of the physiological and structural elements which increase susceptibility to these diseases. Postponement of various degenerative processes would have enhanced benefits because the manifestations increase
exponentially. We need only to learn of individual mechanisms to maintain bone integrity, the retina, the cochlea, and
the various chemical and structural elements of the brain to

gain precious years of comfortable aging. The approach, of course, is not revolutionary, but by the same token, it is not one that is customarily followed. We propose to alter priorities with the goal of postponing events rather than achieving a total cure and particularly for diseases which do not kill but only compromise.

REFERENCES

Abraham S, Johnson CL, & Najjar MF. Weight by height and age of adults 18–74 years. United States, Vital and Health Statistics, No. 14, US Government Printing Office, Washington DC, 1-12:1977.

Annual Summary of Births, Marriages, Divorces, and Deaths: United States, 1991. Monthly Vital Statistics Report, Vol. 40, No. 13, September 20, 1992.

Bacon WE, & Smith GS. Geographic variation in the occurrence of hip fracture among the elderly population in the United States. *American Journal of Public Health.* In press.

Boyce WJ, & Vessey MP. Rising incidence of fracture of the proximal femur. *The Lancet.*;1:150–151. (1985).

Brock DB, & Brody JA. Statistical and epidemiologic characteristics of the United States elderly population. In: Andres R, Bierman EL, and Hazzard, WR (Eds.). *Principles of Geriatric Medicine.* McGraw-Hill, New York, 1984. pp. 51–71.

Brody JA. The best of times/the worst of times: Aging and dependency in the 21st Century. In: Spicker SF, Ingman, SR, and Lawson, IR (Eds.). *Ethical Dimensions of Geriatric Care.* Holland/ Boston: D. Reidel Publishing Co., 1987. pp. 3–21.

Brody JA. Changing health needs of the aging population. Proceedings of the CIBA Foundation Symposium No. 134: Research and the Aging Population, John Wiley & Sons, pp. 208–215. (1988).

Brody JA. Chronic diseases and disorders: An hypothesis suggesting an age-dependent vs. an age-related class. In: Goldstein, AL (Ed.). *Biomedical Advances in Aging.* New York: Plenum Publishing Corp., pp. 137–142. (1990).

Brody JA. Ha-Ha epidemiology and the compression of morbidity in the aged. *Journal of Clinical Experimental Gerontology.*;4(3):227–38. (1982).

Brody JA. Limited importance of cancer and of competing-risk theories in aging. *Journal Clinical Experimental Gerontology*;5(2)141–54. (1983).

Brody JA. Prospects for an ageing population. *Nature.*;315;(6) 463–466. (1985).

Brody JA, Farmer ME, & White LR. Absence of menopausal effect on hip fracture occurrence in white females. *American Journal of Public Health*;74(12) 1397–1398. (1984).

Brody JA, Freels S, & Miles TP. Epidemiological issues in the developed world. The Ageing of Populations and Communities, In: *Oxford Textbook of Geriatric Medicine.* Oxford University Press; 14–20. (1992).

Brody JA, & Miles TP. Mortality postponed and the unmasking of age-dependent non-fatal conditions. *Aging*;2(3):283–289. (1990).

Brody JA, & Schneider EL. Diseases and disorders of aging: An hypothesis. *Journal of Chronic Disease.*;39(11)871–876. (1986).

Carey JR, Liedo P, Orozco D, & Vaupel JW. Slowing of Mortality Rates at Older Ages in Large Medfly Cohorts. *Science,* 258:457–460, (1992).

Crimmins E. Life Expectancy and the Older Population: Demographic Implications of Recent and Prospective Trends in Old Age Mortality. *Research on Aging,* 6(4):490–514. (1984).

Demographic Yearbook. Pub. No. ST/ESA/STAT/SER.R/16 New York. United Nations, 1986.

Dunn JE, Rudberg MA, Furner SE, & Cassel CK. Mortality Disability, and Falls in Older Persons: The Role of Underlying Disease and Disability. *American Journal of Public Health*; 82:3:395. (1992).

Ewbank D, & Wray JD. Population and public health, in Maxcy-Rosenau(ed.), *Public Health and Prevention Medicine,* 11th ed., Appleton-Century-Crofts, New York, 1504–1548. (1980).

Farmer ME, White LR, Brody JA, & Bailey KR. Race and sex differences in hip fracture incidence. *American Journal of Public Health,*74 (123) 1374–1380. (1984).

Finch CE. *Longevity, Senescence, and the Genome.* The University of Chicago Press, 1990.

Fries JF. Aging, natural death, and the compression of morbidity. *New England Journal of Medicine.*;303:130–135. (1980).

Gosden RG. *Biology of menopause: The causes and consequences of ovarian ageing.* Academic Press, London. (1985).

Guralnik JM, LaCroix AZ, Everett DF, & Kovar MG. Aging in the Eighties: The Prevalence of Comorbidity and Its Association with Disability. Advance Data. Vital and Health Statistics of the National Center for Health Statistics. US Department of Health and Human Services, Public Health Service Centers for Disease Control No. 170, 1989.

Herrick JB Clinical features of sudden obstruction of the coronary arteries, *The Journal of the American Medical Association;* 59:2015–2020, (1912).

Hume D. An enquiry concerning human understanding. In *Encyclopedia Britannica;* 491. Chicago, London, Toronto. (1952).

Kimura N. The rising pandemic of mental disorders and associated chronic diseases, stroke, and nutrient intake in Japan, *Preventive Medicine;* 12:222–227, (1983).

Kellie SE, & Brody JA. Sex- and race-specific hip fracture rates. *American Journal of Public Health;*80(3):326–328. (1990).

Kimura N. Changing patterns of coronary heart disease, stroke, and nutrient intake in Japan, *Preventive Medicine;* 12:222–227. (1983).

Kinsella K. Aging in the Third World, International Population Reports Series, 95, No. 79, U.S. Government Printing Office, Washington DC. (1993).

Manton K, Larry SC, & Stallard E. Changes in the Use of Personal Assistance and Special Equipment. 1982–1989:Results from the 1982 and 1989 National Long Term Care Survey. *The Gerontologist.* In press.

Manton KG, Stallard E, & Tolley HD. Limits to Human Life Expectancy. *Population and Development;* 17(4):603–637. (Rev. 1991).

Meyers G, & Manton K. Compression of Mortality: Myth or Reality? *Gerontologist;* 24:346–353. (1984).

Miles TP, & Brody JA. Aging as a worldwide phenomenon. DE Crews and RM Garutto Ed., in press.

National Center for Health Statistics: 1964, The Change in Mortality Trends in the U.S., Series 4, No.1, Washington, D.C.: U.S. Government Printing Office.

Olshansky SJ, Carnes BA, & Cassel CK. The aging of the human species. *Scientific American;* 50–57. (1993).

Olshansky SJ, Rudberg MA, Carnes BA, Cassel CK, & Brody JA.

Trading off longer life for worsening health: The expansion of morbidity hypothesis. *Journal of Aging and Health.*;3(2):194–216. (1990).

Paffenbarger RS, Hyde RT, Wing AL, Lee IM, Jung DL, & Kampert JB. The association of changes in physical-activity level and other lifestyle characteristics with mortality among men, *The England Journal of Medicine*; 328(8): 538–545. (1993).

Rosenberg HM, Klebba AJ, Havlik RJ, & Feinleib M. (Eds.), Proceedings of the Conference on the Decline in Coronary Heart Disease Mortality, NIH Pub. No. 79–1610, U.S. Government Printing Office, Washington, D.C. 11–39, (1979).

Schneider EL, & Brody JA. Aging, natural death and the compression of morbidity: Another view. *New England Journal of Medicine.*;309(14)854–856. (1983).

Stallones RA. The rise and fall of ischemic heart disease. *Scientific American* 243, 53–59. (1982).

Sutherland JE, Persky VW, & Brody JA. Proportionate mortality trends: 1950–1986. *Journal of American Medical Association.*;264(24):3178–3184. (1990).

Torrey BB, Kinsella K, & Taeuber CM. An ageing world international Population Reports Series, 95, No. 78, U.S. Government Printing Office. Washington DC. (1987).

US Department of Health and Human Services, Aging America: Trends and Projects. DHHS Publication No. (FCoA) 91–28001.

United States National Center for Health Statistics. (1991). Changing Mortality Patterns, Health Services Utilization, and Health Care Expenditures. United States, 1978–2003. Hyattsville, Maryland, NCHS Analytical and Epidemiological Studies, Vital and Health Statistics, Series 3, No. 23, DHHS publication No. (PHS)83–1407). (1983).

Welin L, Larsson B, Svardsudd K, Wilhelmsen L, & Tibblin G. Why is the incidence of ischemic heart disease in Sweden increasing?. *American Journal of Public Health*; 71:461–463. (1981).

Zetterberg C, Elmerson S, & Anderson GBJ. Epidemiology of hip fractures in Goteborg, Sweden. *Clinical Orthopedics*;191:43–51, (1940–1983).

Exercise in the Prevention of Age-Associated Changes in Body Composition and Functional Capacity

3

William J. Evans

The sixth age shifts
Into the lean and slipper'd pantaloon,
With spectacles on nose and pouch on side,
His youthful hose, well sav'd, a world too wide
For his shrunk shank; and his big manly voice,
Turning again toward childish treble, pipes
And whistles in his sound. Last scene of all,
That ends this strange eventful history,
Is second childishness and mere oblivion,
Sans teeth, sans eyes, sans taste, sans every thing

(*As You Like It*, Act II, Scene VII, 157–166)

In the 16th century when William Shakespeare wrote these lines, the prevailing notion was that frailty and debility were the natural and inevitable consequences of aging. Unfortunately these ideas have survived to the present.

Certainly we all change as we grow older. And clearly the modifications in function and body composition—chief among them being a substantial reduction in skeletal muscle mass which we have termed *sarcopenia*—that accompany advancing years may in turn increase the risk of many chronic

35

diseases. That these changes are a consequence of *normal* aging has recently been challenged by a number of investigators. This chapter will focus on the causes of sarcopenia and reduced functional capacity and their consequences. We will also present strategies for preventing sarcopenia or reversing its impact.

BODY COMPOSITION

Using total body potassium as an index of fat free mass, Novak (1972) assessed the body composition of more than 500 men and women between the ages of 18 and 85. He determined that body fat increased from 18% to 36% and 33% to 44% in men and women, respectively. In an 18-year longitudinal study, Flynn and coworkers found that the most *rapid* rate of total body potassium loss occurred between the ages of 41 and 60 years for men and not until after the age of 60 in women. Cohn and coworkers (1980), using total body neutron activation procedures, determined that the principal component of the decline in fat free mass was a decrease in muscle mass, with minimal change in nonmuscle mass. They also observed that total body nitrogen declined in very close association with total body calcium, suggesting a link between sarcopenia and osteopenia. Skeletal muscle is the largest reservoir of protein in the body. Age-related reductions in muscle is a direct cause of the age-related decrease in muscle strength (Bruce et al., 1989; Frontera et al., 1991; Larsson et al., 1979; Rice et al., 1989; Young et al., 1984)

Loss of muscle mass with age in humans has been demonstrated both indirectly and directly. The excretion of urinary creatinine, reflecting muscle creatine content and total muscle mass, decreases by nearly 50% between the ages of 20 and 90 (Tzankoff & Norris, 1978) (Fig. 3.1). Computed tomography of individual muscles shows that after age 30, there is a decrease in cross-sectional areas of the thigh along with decreased muscle density associated with increased intramuscular fat. These changes are most pronounced in women (Imamura et al., 1983).

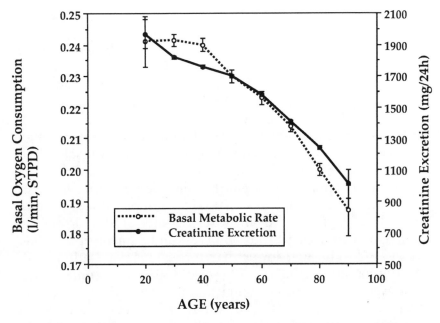

FIGURE 3.1 Reductions in total muscle mass (estimated from creatinine excretion) and resting oxygen consumption indicates the close relationship between these two variables. (Redrawn from Tzankoff & Norris, 1978.)

Muscle atrophy may result from a gradual and selective loss of muscle fibers. The number of muscle fibers in the midsection of the vastus lateralis of autopsy specimens is lower by about 110,000 in elderly men (age 70–73) than in young men (age 19–37), a 23% difference (Lexell et al., 1983). The decline is more marked in Type II muscle fibers, which fall from an average 60% in sedentary young men to below 30% after the age of 80 (Larsson, 1983), and is significantly related to age-related decreases in strength ($r = 0.54$, $P < 0.001$).

A reduction in muscle strength is a major component of normal aging. Data from the Framingham study (Jette & Branch, 1981) indicate that 40% of the female population aged 55 to 64, almost 45% of women aged 65 to 74, and 65% of women aged 75 to 84 years were unable to lift 4.5 kg. In addition, a similarly high percentage of women in this population reported that they were unable to perform some aspects of normal household work. Larsson and colleagues (1979) studied 114 men between the ages of 11 and 70 years and found that isometric and dynamic strength of the quadriceps increased up to the age of 30 years, and decreased after the age of 50. They saw reductions in strength ranging from 24–36% between the ages of 50 and 70 and concluded that much of this was due to a selective atrophy of Type II muscle fibers which were 36% smaller in diameter when compared to 40-year-olds. It appears, though, that muscle strength losses are most dramatic after age of 70. For example, knee extensor strength of a group of healthy 80-year-olds studied in the Copenhagen City Heart Study (Danneskoild-Samsoe et al., 1984) was found to be 30% lower than a previous population study (Aniansson et al., 1981) of 70-year-old men and women. Thus cross-sectional as well as longitudinal data indicate that muscle strength declines by approximately 15% per decade in the 6th and 7th decade and about 30% thereafter (Danneskoild-Samsoe et al., 1984; Harries & Bassey, 1990; Larsson, 1978; Murray et al., 1985). While there is some indication that muscle *function* is reduced with advancing age, the overwhelming majority of the loss in strength results from an age-related decrease in muscle *mass*.

We examined (Frontera et al., 1991) more that 200 men and women between the ages of 45 and 78 years old. Isokinetic and isometric strength of the upper and lower body were significantly different between men and women and both declined with advancing age. However, when corrected for fat-free mass (estimated from hydrostatic weighing) and total body muscle mass (estimated from 24-hour urinary creatinine), age-related differences disappear (Table 3.1).

STRENGTH AND FUNCTIONAL CAPACITY

Bassey, Bendall, and Pearson (1988) measured muscle strength and the amount and speed of customary walking in a

TABLE 3.1 Strength Corrected for Body Composition in Older Women

Age (years)	Strength (Nm)	Nm / FFM	Nm / muscle mass
45–54	108 ± 22	2.7 ± 0.4	6.1 ± 0.9
55–64	98 ± 20	2.6 ± 0.4	5.9 ± 1.2
65–78	89 ± 15*	2.5 ± 0.4	5.8 ± 1.1

*different from age 45–54 group (P < 0.05)
(*Source*: Frontera et al., 1991)

large sample of men and women older than 65 years. They found an age-related decline in muscle strength and a significant negative correlation between strength and chosen normal walking speed for both sexes ($r = 0.041$, $p < 0.001$ for men; $r = 0.36$, $p < 0.01$ for women). Bassey and coworkers (Bassey et al., 1989) measured flexibility and found that the mean value for the elderly was 30 degrees less than those accepted for younger men and women. Nearly one-half of the distribution fell below the accepted threshold level of 120 degrees for adequate function. Fiatarone and collegues observed a closer relationship between quadriceps strength and habitual gait speed ($r = -0.745$, $p < 0.01$) in a group of frail institutionalized men and women above the age of 86 years. In these subjects, fat free mass ($r = 0.732$) and regional muscle mass estimated by computerized tomography ($r = 0.752$) were correlated with muscle strength.

In the same population, we (Bassey et al., 1992) recently demonstrated that leg power—which represents a more dynamic measurement of muscle function—may be a useful predictor of functional capacity in the very old. In older, frail women, for example, leg power was highly correlated with walking speed ($r = 0.93$, $p < 0.001$), accounting for up to 86% of the variance in this activity. These data suggest that with the advancing age and very low activity levels seen in institutionalized patients, muscle strength is a critical component of walking ability.

Further work shows similar results. Whipple, Wolfson, and Amerman (1987) examined nursing home residents and found a significant reduction in strength in all the muscle groups of the knees and ankles in a group of elderly fallers compared with nonfallers. In another study, Blake and coworkers (1988) examined 1,042 home-dwelling men and women older than age 65. Of this sample, 35% reported one or more falls in the preceding year, and among a host of factors that distinguished fallers from nonfallers, such as polypharmacy and arthritis, handgrip strength of the dominant hand emerged as the most important factor. Indeed, handgrip strength has been shown to be predictive of lower extremity strength (Tornvall, 1963). Indeed, all of these studies indicate that muscle weakness becomes an increasingly important component of functional capacity with increasing age.

ENERGY METABOLISM

Daily energy expenditure also declines progressively throughout adult life (McGandy et al., 1966). In sedentary individuals, the main determinant of energy expenditure is fat-free mass (Ravussin et al., 1986), which decreases by about 15% between the third and eighth decade of life, contributing to a lower basal metabolic rate in the elderly (Cohn et al., 1980). Tzankoff and Norris (1978) saw that 24-hour creatinine excretion (an index of muscle mass) was closely related to basal metabolic rate at all ages. Nutrition surveys of those over the age of 65 years show a very low energy intake for men (1400 kcal/day; 23 kcal/kg/day). These data indicate that preservation of muscle mass and prevention of sarcopenia can help prevent the decrease in metabolic rate.

While body weight increases with advancing age, an age-associated increase in relative body fat content has been demonstrated by a number of investigators. The cause of this increase in body fatness results from a number of factors, but chief among these causes are a declining metabolic rate and activity level coupled with an energy intake that does not match this declining need for calories. Meredith et al. demon-

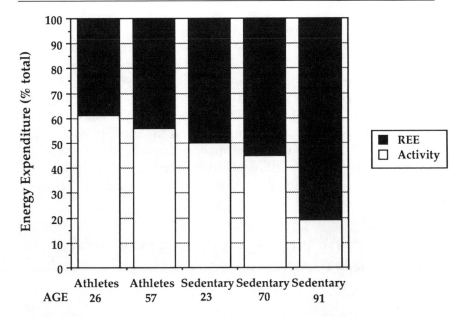

FIGURE 3.2 The above figure is an estimate of the relative contribution of activity and resting energy expenditure in young and middle-aged athletes (bars 1 & 2, Meredith et al., 1987), young and old sedentary men (bars 3 & 4, Roberts et al., 1992), and very old nursing home patients (bar 5, Fiatarone, unpublished data).

strated that endurance-trained men between 20 and 60 years old consumed a diet very high in calories, but that body fat levels were closely related to the total number of hours spent exercising per week. Age was not found to be a covariate in this study. More recently, Roberts and coworkers (1992) examined the relationship between total energy use (using the doubly labeled water technique) and body composition in a group of sedentary young and old men and found that energy spent in daily activity accounted for 73% of the variability in body fat content. Using data published from our laboratory, Figure 3.2 shows the percentage of total daily energy expenditure from daily activities and resting energy expenditure in young and middle-age athletes, young and older sedentary men, and very old nursing home residents.

In addition to its role in energy metabolism, skeletal muscle and its age-related decline may contribute to such age-associated changes as reduction in bone density (Bevier et al.,
1989; Sinaki et al., 1986; Snow-Harter et al., 1990), insulin sensitivity (Kolterman et al., 1980), and aerobic capacity (Flegg &
Lakatta, 1988). For these reasons strategies for preservation
of muscle mass with advancing age and for increasing muscle
mass and strength in the previously sedentary elderly may be
an important way to increase functional independence and
decrease the prevalence of many age-associated chronic
diseases.

CAPACITY OF THE ELDERLY TO RESPOND TO EXERCISE TRAINING

Aerobic Exercise

Maximal aerobic capacity has been demonstrated to decrease at the rate of approximately 1%/year. This decline is
due to a number of factors including decreased maximal cardiac output, decreased muscle mass (Flegg & Lakatta, 1988),
and the decreased oxidative capacity of skeletal muscle
(Meredith et al., 1989). The average VO_{2max} or aerobic capacity
of sedentary 75–80-year-old men and women compared to the
oxygen cost of a number of activities of daily living are shown
in Figure 3.3. As these tasks represent a larger and larger percentage of maximum aerobic capacity, it is not difficult to see
why many elderly (particularly women because of a lower fitness level at all ages) choose not to perform them. The capacity of elderly men and women to respond to increased levels
of physical activity with improvements in strength and/or aerobic capacity depend, in large measure, on the frequency, intensity, and duration of the exercise program. With aerobic
exercise training, intensity is generally reported as a percentage of VO_{2max} or of maximal heart rate. Aerobic training involves high repetition muscle contractions and leads to mini-

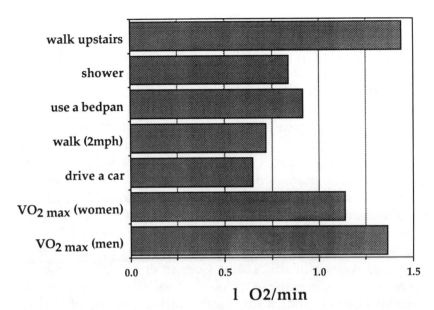

FIGURE 3.3 The average maximal rate of oxygen consumption VO_{2max} in sedentary men and women between 75 and 80 years old compared to the oxygen cost of a number of daily activities.

mal strength gains. Intensity of resistance training is generally reported as a percentage of the one repetition maximum (1 RM), the maximum amount of force that a muscle group can generate with one single contraction.

A number of studies have shown a great capacity of the elderly to respond to aerobic exercise. A study (Seals et al., 1984b) examining the effects of 6 months of low intensity and 6 months of high intensity exercise demonstrated that healthy 60–70-year-old subjects increased their average VO_{2max} by 30% with a range of 2%–49%. There was no change in maximal cardiac output as a result of the year long intervention, but a decrease in blood lactate levels during a standard exercise task was observed. The authors concluded that the increase in maximal aerobic capacity occurred as a result of peripheral rather than central adaptations.

Our laboratory (Meredith et al., 1989) compared the peripheral effects of vigorous endurance exercise (stationary cycling: 45 min/day, 3 days/wk at 70% of maximal heart rate reserve) in young (24-year-old) and older (65-year-old) men and women. The muscle oxidative capacity (from *m. vastus lateralis* biopsies) of the older subjects increased by an average of 128% while the young subjects showed only a 27% increase. The absolute increase in VO_{2max} was not different between the two groups, however the relative improvement in the older subjects was 20% versus 12% in the younger subjects. Kohrt and coworkers examined the adaptations of 53 men and 57 women between the ages of 60 and 71 years to 9–12 months of regular aerobic exercise (walk/run: 4 days/wk, 45 min/day, 80% maximal heart rate). They observed an average 24% increase in VO_{2max} with a large range (0–58%). In a subset of 23 men and women in this study, Coggan et al. (1992) observed large increases in muscle mitochondrial enzyme activity and capillary density indicating a substantial capacity of skeletal muscle to respond to regular aerobic exercise.

Aging is associated with decreased glucose tolerance and a greatly increased incidence of non-insulin dependent diabetes mellitus (NIDDM). This waning glucose tolerance can lead to the previously mentioned age-associated changes in body composition and activity levels (Kolterman et al., 1980). Improved fitness as a result of aerobic exercise has also been demonstrated to improve glucose tolerance in previously sedentary subjects (Holloszy et al., 1986; Seals et al., 1984a) and exercise has been shown to prevent the onset of NIDDM (Helmrich et al., 1991).

Recently, our laboratory (Hughes et al., 1993) examined the effects of 12 weeks of high or low intensity aerobic exercise (cycle ergometry: 4 days/wk, 45 min/day at 55% or 75% of maximal heart rate) with no weight loss on aspects of muscle and whole body carbohydrate metabolism. Men and women with impaired glucose tolerance were selected for participation after an oral glucose tolerance test. No differences were seen between the low- and high-intensity exercise. Significant improvements in oral glucose tolerance and insulin-stimulated glucose disposal rate were accompanied by increased skeletal muscle glycogen levels and a 68% increase in muscle GLUT–4 levels. These data indicate that improvements in carbohydrate metabolism resulting from exercise occur primarily in skeletal muscle. By increasing the opportunity for body fat loss as well as stimulating the adaptive response of skeletal muscle which is the primary site of glucose disposal, exercise can clearly improve glucose metabolism not only in diabetics but in people at high risk for developing NIDDM as well.

Strength Training

Strength conditioning is training in which the resistance against which a muscle generates force is progressively increased over time, resulting in an increase in muscle size. It is clear that elderly subjects achieve only modest increases in strength when the intensity of the exercise is low (Aniansson & Gustafsson, 1981; Larsson, 1982). A number of studies have demonstrated, though, that given an adequate training stimulus, older men and women show similar or greater strength gains compared to young individuals as a result of resistance training.

Frontera et al. (1988; 1990) showed that older men responded to a 12-week Progressive Resistance Training (PRT) program (80% of the 1 repetition maximum, 3 sets of 8 repetitions of the knee extensor and flexors, 3 days per week) by more than doubling extensor strength and more than tripling flexor strength. The increases in strength averaged approximately 5% per training session, similar to strength gains observed by younger men. Total muscle area estimated by computerized tomography (CT) increased by 11.4%. Biopsies of the vastus lateralis muscle revealed similar increases in type I fiber area (33.5%) and type II fiber area (27.6%). Daily excretion of urinary 3-methyl-L-histidine increased with training ($P < 0.05$) by an average of 40.8%, indicating that increased muscle size and strength resulting from PRT are associated

TABLE 3.2 Effects of Strength Training on Determinants of VO_{2max}

	Week 0	Week 12
VO_{2max} (leg ergometry)		
1 / min	2.07 ±0.07	2.19 ±0.08*
ml • kg FFM^{-1} • min^{-1}	38.6 ±1.2	40.5 ±1.6*
VO_{2max} (leg ergometry)		
1 / min	1.41 ±0.05	1.41 ±0.06
ml • kg FFM^{-1} • min^{-1}	26.2 ±0.9	26.2 ±1.0
Mean muscle fiber area, mm2	4,517 ±315	5,435 ±115*
Capillaries / fiber	1.41 ±0.05	1.60 ±1.1*
Citrate synthase activity		
mmol • g-1 • min-1	9.6 ±1.1	13.1 ±1.1*

* significantly different from week 0 ($P < 0.05$)
(*Source*: Frontera et al., 1990)

with an increased rate of myofibrillar protein turnover. In these subjects, the effects of PRT on maximal aerobic power (VO_{2max}) was also measured. Leg cycle ergometer VO_{2max} increased by an average 1.9 ml/kg lean body mass/minute ($P = 0.034$) while arm cycle VO_{2max} was unchanged. Biopsies of the vastus lateralis showed significant increases in capillary density (Table 3.2) and citrate synthase activity, suggesting that high intensity strength training can result in increased oxidative capacity of the muscles being exercised. Another possible explanation is that as a result of increasing leg strength, the subjects in this study increased their activity levels, thus increasing aerobic capacity. Whatever its cause, the increase in leg VO_{2max} resulted from increased muscle mass and oxidative capacity. Charette et al. examined the effects of 12 weeks of resistance training (65–75% of 1 RM) in older women and also demonstrated substantial increases in leg muscle strength along with a 20% increase in type II muscle fiber area.

The very old and frail elderly experience skeletal muscle atrophy as a result of disuse, disease, undernutrition, and the effects of aging, per se. In addition, muscle weakness that accompanies advanced age increases the risk of falling and fracture in these older individuals (Scheibel, 1985). For this reason we chose a group of institutionalized elderly men and women (age range 87–96 years) in order to study the effects of high-intensity, progressive resistance training on quadriceps muscle strength. Not surprisingly, initial strength levels were extremely low in these subjects, with a mean 1 RM of 8 kg for the quadriceps. The absolute amount of weight lifted by the subjects during the training increased from 8 to 21 kg. The results were dramatic. Average increase in strength after 8 weeks of resistance training was $174 \pm 31\%$ and mean increase in muscle cross-sectional area via computerized tomography was $10 \pm 8\%$. The substantial increases in muscle size and strength were accompanied by clinically significant improvements in tandem gait speed, and index of functional mobility. Repeat 1 RM testing in seven of the subjects after 4 weeks of no training showed that quadriceps strength had declined 32%.

This study demonstrates that frail elderly men and women, well into their 10th decade of life, retain the capacity to adapt to progressive resistance exercise training with significant and clinically relevant muscle hypertrophy and increases in muscle strength. Results from the resistance training studies performed in young, middle-age, elderly, and the oldest old indicate that it is the intensity of the stimulus, not the underlying fitness or frailty of the individual, that determines the magnitude of the gains in strength and muscle size.

In conclusion, sarcopenia, defined as the age-related loss in skeletal muscle mass, results in decreased strength and aerobic capacity and thus functional capacity. Sarcopenia is also closely linked to age-related losses in bone mineral, basal metabolic rate and increased body fat content. Through physical exercise and training, primarily resistance training, it may be possible to prevent sarcopenia and the remarkable array of associated abnormalities, such as NIDDM, coronary artery disease, hypertension, osteoporosis, and obesity. Using an exercise program of sufficient frequency, intensity, and duration, it is quite possible to increase muscle strength and endurance at any age. Indeed, there is no pharmacological intervention that holds a greater promise of improving health and promoting independence in the elderly than does exercise. After all, even Shakespeare centuries ago recognized that aging did not necessarily have to be associated with frailty and that functional capacity in old age was a result of lifestyle rather than chronology:

> Be comfort to my age! Here is the gold
> All this I give you. Let me be your servant.
> Though I look old, yet I am strong and lusty;
> For in my youth I never did apply
> Hot and rebellious liquors in my blood,
> Nor did not with unbashful forehead woo
> The means of weakness and debility;
> Therefore my age is as a lusty winter,
> Frosty, but kindly. Let me go with you;
> I'll do the service of a younger man
> In all your business and necessities.

> (*As You Like It*, Act II, Scene III, 44–55)

REFERENCES

Aniansson, A., Grimby, G., Hedberg, M., & Krotkiewski, M. (1981). Muscle morphology, enzyme activity and muscle strength in elderly men and women. *Clin. Physiol., 1*, 73–86.

Aniansson, A., & Gustafsson, E. (1981). Physical training in elderly men with special reference to quadriceps muscle strength and morphology. *Clin. Physiol., 1*, 87–98.

Bassey, E. J., Bendall, M. J., & Pearson, M. (1988). Muscle strength in the triceps surae and objectively measured customary walking activity in men and women over 65 years of age. *Clin. Sci., 74*, 85–89.

Bassey, E. J., Fiatarone, M. A., O'Neill, E. F., Kelly, M., Evans, W. J., & Lipsitz, L. A. (1992). Leg extensor power and functional performance in very old men and women. *Clin. Sci., 82*, 321–327.

Bassey, E. J., Morgan, K., Dallosso, H. M., et al. (1989). Flexibility of the shoulder joint measured as a range of abduction in a large representative sample of men and women over 65 years of age. *Eur. J. Appl. Physiol., 58*, 353–360.

Bevier, W. C., Wiswell, R. A., Pyka, G., Kozak, K. C., Newhall, K. M., & Marcus, R. (1989). Relationship of body composition, muscle strength, and aerobic capacity to bone mineral density in older men and women. *J. Bone Min. Res., 4*, 421–432.

Blake, A. J., Morgan, K., & Bendall, M. J. (1988). Falls by elderly people at home: Prevalence and associated factors. *Age Ageing, 17*, 365–372.

Bruce, S. A., Newton, D., & Woledge, R. C. (1989). Effect of age on voluntary force and cross-sectional area of human adductor possicis muscle. *Q. J. Exp. Physiology, 74*, 359–362.

Coggan, A. R., Spina, R. J., King, D. S., Rogers, M. A., Brown, M., Nemeth, P. M., & Holloszy, J. O. (1992). Skeletal muscle adaptations to endurance training in 60- to 70-yr-old men and women. *J. Appl. Physiol., 72*, 1780–1786.

Cohn, S. H., Vartsky, D., Yasumura, S., Savitsky, A., Zanzi, I., Vaswani, A., & Ellis, K. J. (1980). Compartmental body composition based on total-body, potassium, and calcium. *Am. J. Physiol., 239*, E524-E530.

Danneskoild-Samsoe, B., Kofod, V., Munter, J., Grimby, G., Schnohr, P., & Jensen, G. (1984). Muscle strength and functional capacity in 77–81-year-old men and women. *Eur. J. Appl. Physiol., 52*.

Flegg, J. L., & Lakatta, E. G. (1988). Role of muscle loss in the age-associated reduction in VO2max. *J. Appl. Physiol., 65*, 1147–1151.

Frontera, W. R., Hughes, V. A., & Evans, W. J. (1991). A cross-sectional study of upper and lower exeremity muscle strength in 45–78-year-old men and women. *J. Appl. Physiol., 71*, 644–650.

Frontera, W. R., Meredith, C. N., O'Reilly, K. P., & Evans, W. J. (1990). Strength training and determinants of VO_{2max} in older men. *J. Appl. Physiol., 68*, 329–333.

Frontera, W. R., Meredith, C. N., O'Reilly, K. P., Knuttgen, H. G., & Evans, W. J. (1988). Strength conditioning in older men: skeletal muscle hypertrophy and improved function. *J. Appl. Physiol., 64*, 1038–1044.

Harries, U. J., & Bassey, E. J. (1990). Torque-velocity relationships for the knee extensors in women in their 3rd and 7th decades. *Eur. J. Appl. Physiol., 60*, 187–190.

Helmrich, S. P., Ragland, D. R., Leung, R. W., & Paffenbarger, R. S. (1991). Physical activity and reduced occurrence of non-insulin-dependent diabetes mellitus. *N. Engl. J. Med., 325*, 147–152.

Holloszy, J. O., Schultz, J., Kusnierkiewicz, J., Hagberg, J. M., & Ehsani, A. A. (1986). Effects of exercise on glucose tolerance and insulin resistance. *Acta Med. Scand. (Suppl.)*, *711*, 55–65.

Hughes, V. A., Fiatarone, M. A., Fielding, R. A., Kahn, B. B., Ferra, C. M., Shepherd, P., Fisher, E. C., Wolfe, R. R., Elahi, D., & Evans, W. J. (1993). Exercise increases muscle GLUT 4 levels and insulin in subjects with impaired glucose tolerance. *Am. J. Physiol.*, *264*, E855-E862.

Imamura, K., Ashida, H., Ishikawa, T., & Fujii, M. (1983). Human major psoas muscle and scrospinalis muscle in relation to age: A study by computed tomography. *J. Gerontol.*, *38*, 678–681.

Jette, A. M., & Branch, L. G. (1981). The Framingham disability study: II. Physical disability among the aging. *Am. J. Public Health*, *71*, 1211–1216.

Kolterman, O. G., Insel, J., Saekow, M., & Olefsky, J. M. (1980). Mechanisms of insulin resistance in human obesity. Evidence for receptor and postreceptor defects. *J. Clin. Invest.*, *65*, 1272–1284.

Larsson, L. (1978). Morphological and functional characteristics of the ageing skeletal muscle in man. *Acta Physiol. Scand. Suppl.*, *457*, 1–36.

Larsson, L. (1982). Physical training effects on muscle morphology in sedentary males as different ages. *Med. Sci. Sports Exercise*, *14*, 203–206.

Larsson, L. (1983). Histochemical characteristics of human skeletal muscle during aging. *Acat Physiol. Scand.*, *117*, 469–471.

Larsson, L. G., Grimby, G., & Karlsson, J. (1979). Muscle strength and speed of movement in relation to age and muscle morphology. *J. Appl. Physiol.*, *46*, 451–456.

Lexell, J., Henriksson-Larsen, K., Wimblod, B., & Sjostrom, M. (1983). Distribution of different fiber types in human skeletal muscles: Effects of aging studied in whole muscle cross sections. *Muscle Nerve*, *6*, 588–595.

MacDougall, J. D. (1986). Adaptability of muscle to strength training—a cellular approach. In B. Saltin (Ed.), *Biochemistry of Exercise IV* (pp. 501–513). Champaing, IL: Human Kinetics.

McGandy, R. B., Barrows, C. H., Spanias, A., Meredith, A., L., S. J., & Norris, A. H. (1966). Nutrient intake and energy expenditure in men of different ages. *J. Gerontol.*, *21*, 581–587.

Meredith, C. N., Frontera, W. R., Fisher, E. C., A., H. V., Herland, J. C., Edwards, J., & Evans, W. J. (1989). Peripheral effects of endurance training in young and old subjects. *J. Appl. Physiol.*, *66*, 2844–2849.

Meredith, C. N., Zackin, M. J., Frontera, W. R., & Evans, W. J. (1987). Body composition and aerobic capacity in young and middle-aged endurance-trained men. *Med. Sci. Sports Exerc.*, *19*, 557–563.

Murray, M. P., Duthie, E. H., Gambert, S. T., Sepic, S. B., & Mollinger, L. A. (1985). Age-related differences in knee muscle strength in normal women. *J. Gerontol.*, *40*, 275–280.

Novak, L. P. (1972). Aging, total body potassium, fat free-mass, and cell mass in males and females between ages 18 and 85 years. *J. Gerontol.*, *24*, 438–459.

Ravussin, E., Lillioja, S., Anderson, T. E., Cristin, L., & Bogardus, C. (1986). Determinants of 24-hour energy expenditure in man. *J. Clin. Invest.*, *78*, 1568–1578.

Rice, C. L., Cunningham, D. A., Paterson, D. H., & Rechnitzer, P. A. (1989). Strength in an elderly population. *Arch. Phys. Med. Rehabil.*, *70*, 391–397.

Roberts, S. B., Young, V. R., Fuss, P., Heyman, M. B., Fiatarone, M., Dallal, G., Cortiella, J., & Evans, W. J. (1992). What are the dietary energy needs of elderly adults? *Int. J. Obesity*, *16*, 969–976.

Scheibel, A. (1985). Falls, motor dysfunction, and correlative neuro-histologic changes in the elderly. *Clin. in Geriatr. Med.*, *1*, 671–677.

Seals, D. R., Hagberg, J. M., Hurley, B. F., Ehsani, A. A., & Holloszy, J. O. (1984a). Effects of endurance training on glucose tolerance and plasma lipid levels in older men and women. *JAMA*, *252*, 645–649.

Seals, D. R., Hagberg, J. M., Hurley, b. F., Ehsani, A. A., & Holloszy, J. O. (1984b). Endurance training on older men and women. I. Cardiovascular response to exercise. *J. Appl Physiol.*, *57*, 1024–1029.

Sinaki, M., McPhee, M. C., & Hodgson, S. F. (1986). Relationship between bone mineral density of spine and strength of back extensors in healthy postmenopausal women. *Mayo Clin. Proc.*, *61*, 116–122.

Snow-Harter, C., Bouxsein, M., Lewis, B., Charette, S., Weinstein, P., & Marcus, R. (1990). Muscle strength as a predictor of bone mineral density in young women. *J. Bone Min. Res.*, *5*, 589–595.

Tornvall, G. (1963). Assessment of physical capabilities with special reference to the evaluation of maximal voluntary isometric muscle strength and maximal working capacity. *Acta Physiol. Scand., 58 (supplement)*, 201, 1–102.

Tzankoff, S. P., & Norris, A. H. (1978). Longitudinal changes in basal metabolic rate in man. *J. Appl. Physiol., 33*, 536–539.

Whipple, R. H., Wolfson, L. I., & Amerman, P. M. (1987). The relationship of knee and ankle weakness to falls in nursing home residents. *J. Am. Geriatr. Soc., 35*, 13–20.

Young, A., Stokes, M., & Crowe, M. (1984). The size and strength of the quadriceps muscle of old and young women. *Eur. J. Clin. Invest., 14*, 282–287.

Aging-Associated Immune Dysfunction and Strategies to Delay Its Onset

4

Norman R. Klinman,

Phyllis-Jean Linton,

and Debra J. Decker

OVERVIEW

The immune system is crucial to the maintenance of health, particularly with respect to defense against pathogens. Among the numerous physiological defects associated with aging is a generalized decrease in immune function which leads to greater susceptibility to infectious agents as well as an increased morbidity and mortality of infectious disease. Aged individuals are also compromised in their response to vaccination further increasing their susceptibility to endemic and pandemic infectious agents.

The immune system is comprised of three general cell types, T cells, B cells, and accessory or antigen presenting cells, and all three are affected by aging. The aspect of the humoral immune response that is most affected by aging is helper T cell (T_H) dependent B cell responses which require the collaborative interaction of cells of all three types. Such T_H dependent B cell re-

53

sponses usually require for their induction the initial uptake of antigen by dendritic cells, macrophages, or other accessory cells. These cells process antigen such that peptides derived from the antigen are presented in a groove of the class II MHC molecules on their surface. These peptide-MHC complexes are recognized by T_H receptor complexes and via this interaction and interactions with other cell surface accessory molecules, the T_H are activated. These activated T_H are then competent to stimulate B cells that present the same peptide in their class II MHC molecules. In aged individuals, the molecular mechanisms responsible for antigen processing and presentation by both accessory cells and B cells remain intact (Perkins et al., 1982); however, the functionality of the T_H compartment is markedly decreased. Because of this, B cell responses and antibody production against numerous pathogens are substantially reduced in aged individuals. Among infectious agents, responses to viral antigens are largely T_H dependent and are thereby the most compromised. For example, although the frequency and responsiveness of influenza specific B cells are not reduced in aged mice, antibody production is greatly reduced because of decreased T_H function (Zharhary & Klinman, 1984).

Aging Associated T Cell Dysfunction

As reported by Miller and others, much of the decrease in T cell function in aged individuals can be attributed to a shift in T cell subsets such that the majority of T cells in aged individuals have the phenotypic characteristics of memory T cells (Rabinowe et al., 1987; Hallgren et al., 1988; De Paoli et al., 1988; Lerner et al., 1989; Ernst et al., 1990; Grossmann et al., 1991, Flurkey et al., 1992). Additionally, as shown in Figure 4.1, these memory type T cells in aged individuals respond less vigorously to various stimuli than do their counterparts in young adults (Lerner et al., 1989). Although it is not clear whether these poorly responsive cells, which accumulate in the aged T cell pool, would respond normally to their cognate antigen (since the

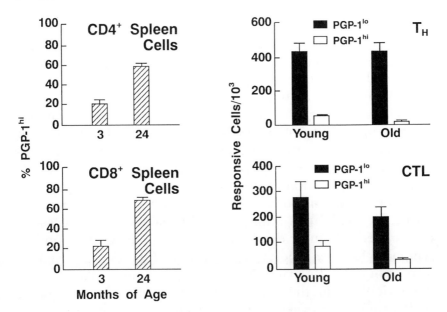

FIGURE 4.1 The percentage of CD4$^{2/3}$ and CD8$^{2/3}$ in 3 and 18 month old mice as determined by FACS analysis is shown in the figures on the left. The frequency of conconavalin A responsive cells among PgP-1^{hi} and PgP-1^{lo} sorted T$_H$ and CTL precursors of aged and young mice as determined by limiting dilution analysis is shown in the figures on the right. It can be seen that the proportion of cells bearing high levels of PgP-1, a characteristic of memory T cells, increases greatly with aging. In addition, the responsiveness of PgP-1^{hi} cells obtained from aged mice is much lower than those of young mice. (Abstracted from Lerner et al., 1989.)

antigen that might have originally induced them is not known), their presence insures that fewer responsive T$_H$ will be available for responses to new antigenic confrontations.

Aging Associated Dysfunction in Memory B Cell Generation

Perhaps the greatest impact of decreased T$_H$ function is found in the generation of B cell memory. While most primary antibody responses are T_H dependent, some antibody responses can be generated T_H independently by direct interaction of antigens with B cells. However, the generation of memory B cells is absolutely dependent on T_H interactions. Since the production of high affinity antibodies which maximize viral inactivation and the success of vaccination are dependent on the generation of memory B cells, the impact of decreased T_H function on this process has severe consequences. In addition to T_H, which are essential for the generation of memory B cells, the propagation of memory responses and the progressive increase in antibody affinity appear also to be dependent on the normal functioning of highly specialized accessory cells called follicular dendritic cells (FDC). FDC are found in lymphoid follicles wherein the germinal centers that give rise to memory B cells originate. FDC provide an antigen retaining reticulum in these locations and antibodies bound on their extended processes bind antigen in a temporally stable fashion (Szakal et al., 1988). In aged mice, the function of these FDC and their ability to generate an antigen retaining reticulum is also compromised (Szakal et al., 1988). It now appears likely that this decrease in FDC function may be secondary to decreased T_H function.

Recent studies from our laboratory have demonstrated that memory B cells are generated from a definable precursor cell subset that is distinct from precursors that generate antibody forming cells (AFC) upon stimulation (Linton et al., 1989). These progenitors of memory B cells can be isolated by their low expression of a cell surface antigen recognized by the J11D monoclonal antibody (J11D^{lo}), and such cells when antigenically stimulated give rise to memory B cells rather than AFC. These J11D^{lo} precursors are also unique in their ability to originate germinal centers (Linton et al., 1992). Analyses of the J11D^{lo} precursor subset in aged mice indicate that they are normal in both frequency and function (Linton, 1993). Therefore, the inability of aged mice to generate normal memory B cell responses is likely to be primarily the result of decreased T_H function (and perhaps decreased FDC function).

Strategies to Delay Aging Associated Dysfunction in T Cells and Memory B Cell Generation

Clearly the aging associated decrease of the immune response to infectious agents and vaccines could be greatly ameliorated if T_H function could be maintained at youthful levels. Several approaches to this goal have been attempted. One approach has been to increase the effectiveness of the remaining functional T_H in aged individuals particularly in conjunction with vaccination. This has been accomplished by the use of adjuvants and cytokines (Thoman & Weigle, 1985; Allison & Byars, 1992). In experimental animals, such efforts have led to better vaccine "takes."

Rather than merely boosting the reactivity of residual functional T cells, other approaches have been to attempt to restore the functionality of the bulk of peripheral T cells in aged individuals or delay the accumulation of dysfunctional T cells through the use of diet or hormones (Frasca et al., 1987; Grossmann et al., 1990; Effros et al., 1991; Chandra, 1992; Cillari et al., 1992). To date, the most impressive results have been reported by the Daynes laboratory using dehydroepiandrosterone sulfate (DHEAS), a precursor to the steroid hormone DHEA (Daynes & Areneo, 1992). As shown in Figure 4.2, treatment with DHEAS appears to increase the number of functional T_H in aged mice, and in so doing appears to increase the humoral immune response to immunization. The efficacy of this approach in humans is currently under investigation. If appropriate hormonal therapy can restore T_H function in the elderly, it could also be used to delay the onset of T_H dysfunction.

Anti-Idiotypic Regulation and Aging

In addition to the aging associated decrease in humoral antibody responses imposed by decreased T_H and FDC function, responses of B cells are further hampered by a broadly specific increase in anti-idiotypic (network) down-regulation. Af-

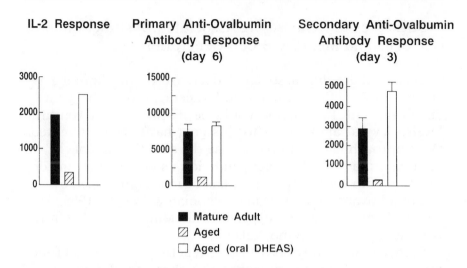

FIGURE 4.2   IL-2 production and primary and secondary antibody responses (as measured in ELISA units) were compared in young mice (13 weeks), aged mice (114 weeks), and aged mice (114 weeks) that had received 100 lg/ml DHEAS in their drinking water for the previous 61 weeks. It can be seen that the aging asociated decrease in responsivenes was obviated by the DHEAS supplementation. (Abstracted from Daynes and Areneo, 1992.)

ter immunization, animals respond not only by producing antibody against the immunizing antigen, but also by generating an immune response which recognizes determinants on the variable regions (idiotypic determinants) of the newly generated antibodies (Rodkey, 1974; Pierce & Klinman, 1977). These anti-idiotypic responses can down-regulate subsequent responses of primary (but not memory) B cells that share these idiotypic determinants. In young animals the generation of anti-idiotypic down-regulation appears to be mainly a consequence of overt immunization. However, aged mice spontaneously display a similar down regulation of B cells specific for numerous antigens (Klinman, 1981; Goidl et al., 1984). Since anti-idiotypic down-regulation following antigenic stimulation is long-lived, it has been reasoned that the antigenic experiences of a lifetime may have generated a broad array of anti-idiotypic responses which accumulate and generally hamper B cell responses of aged individuals.

Aging Associated Alterations in B Cell Function

Although the frequency of B cells responsive to some but not all antigens is somewhat decreased in aged individuals, diversity of the antibody repertoire is not diminished and responsive B cells appear quite normal in their capacity to proliferate and produce antibody (Zharhary & Klinman, 1984; Linton et al., 1989; Zharhary & Klinman, 1986; Zharhary & Klinman, 1986a). The major intrinsic alteration of B cells of aged mice is an unexpected shift in variable region generation (Zharhary & Klinman, 1986b; Riley et al., 1989; Nicoletti et al., 1991; Goidl et al., 1990).

Immunoglobulin variable regions are generated by a complex series of gene rearrangements (see Fig. 4.3). At an early stage in B cell development, a series of enzymes that mediate Ig heavy chain gene segment recombination are expressed. In general, the first rearrangement events involve the rearrangement of one of numerous (13 in the mouse) D_H minigene segments to one of four J_H minigene segments on both chromosomes (Alt et al., 1984). This process can be followed either by a) a further D_H-J_H rearrangement involving an upstream D_H and a downstream J_H splicing out the earlier rearrangement, or b) the rearrangement of a V_H gene segment to a rearranged D_H-J_H. Presumably, due to the propensity for multiple D_H->J_H rearrangements prior to V_H->D_H-J_H, the most upstream J_H (J_{HI}) is underrepresented (10%) in the final V_H-D_H-J_H products and very often it is associated with the most upstream D_H gene segment, DFL16.1 (Teale & Medina, 1992; Feeney, 1990) (i.e., rearrangements of DFL16.1 with J_{HI} could not be displaced by a subsequent D_H->J_H rearrangement event).

In adult bone marrow, precursors of B cells express the enzyme terminal dideoxytransferase (TdT) during the course of H chain gene segment rearrangement (Desiderio et al., 1984). This enzyme adds non-germline encoded nucleotides (N addi-

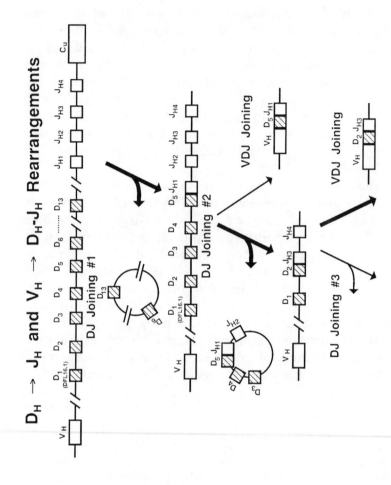

FIGURE 4.3 The events in immunoglobulin H chaim variable rearrangements are diagrammed. Rearrangement of V_H may follow a single or multiple rounds of $D_H > J_H$ rearrangements. (After Alt et al., 1984.)

tions) at the D_H-J_H and V_H-D_H junctions, greatly adding to the extent of diversity in the third complementarity determining region (HCDR3). Indeed, HCDR3 is so diverse in the presence of N additions that any given sequence would not be likely to recur within an individual's lifetime (Decker et al., 1991).

Variable region diversity is further amplified by the combinatorial association of H chains with a diverse set of L chains. L chain rearrangement is generally initiated after H chain expression and clonal expansion. Because there are no D regions and N additions are rare, L chains are less diverse than H chains.

In spite of the enormous potential for diversity in variable regions generated in the adult bone marrow, there are a few clonotypes that are extremely unusual in that all individuals continuously express them in thousands of B cells and re-express them throughout their lifetime. The premier example of such a specificity is the T15 clonotype wherein antibodies with an identical sequence dominate the response of BALB/c mice (and closely related clonotypes in other murine strains) to phosphorylcholine (PC), the dominant antigenic determinant of *Streptococcus (S.) pneumoniae* (Gearhart et al., 1975; Klinman & Stone, 1983; Lieberman et al., 1974; Perlmutter et al., 1984).

It is in this particular response that altered repertoire expression in aged mice was first identified. The T15 antibody which represents over 80% of the response to PC of young adult mice, requires a single light chain (K_{T15}-Jj_5) and an H chain V region comprised of V_1 (a member of the V_HS107 family) joined at a precise nucleotide with DFL16.1 which is joined precisely with J_{H1}. In aged mice, the frequency of T15$^+$ B cells is increased. In addition, superimposed on this response is a spectrum of PC specific B cells that utilize variable region genes rarely found in PC responses of young adult mice (Zharhary & Klinman, 1986b; Riley et al., 1989; Nicoletti et al., 1991). By analyzing the PC specific repertoire of newly generated bone marrow cells, we were able to fully analyze these specificities and demonstrate that the alteration in aged mice was at the level of repertoire generation. This analysis is presented in Figure 4.4. It can be seen that among newly generated B cells the frequency of T15$^+$ B cells is

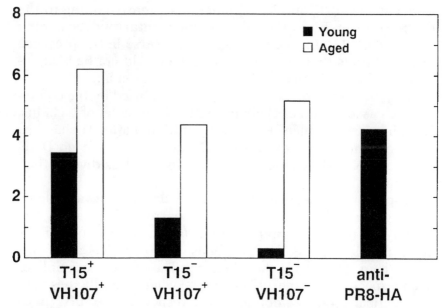

FIGURE 4.4 The frequency of newly generated bone marrow B cells expressing anti-PC antibodies of various phenotypes in aged vs. young mice. It can be seen that all three phenotypes are increased in aging particularly those which are extremely rare in young adults. The last column presents the frequency of bone marrow cells responsive to all determinants of an influenza virus hemmaglutinin for purposes of comparison. (Abstracted from Riley et al., 1989.)

increased twofold in aged mice. PC responsive B cells that use the same V_H gene segment (or a closely related gene segment) but do not share sequence in other regions (D_H, J_H, or L chain) with T15, while infrequent in young adults, are prevalent in aged mice. Most dramatic is the appearance of large numbers of PC responsive B cells in aged mice that utilize V_H gene segments other than a member of the V_HS107 family. Such B cells are extremely rare in young adults.

Does this alteration of repertoire have any implications for protection against bacterial pathogens? In a recent series of experiments, the laboratory of Dr. Jan Cerny has analyzed the protection of mice against *S. pneumoniae* pathogenesis using various passively transferred antibodies (Nicoletti et al., 1993). Their findings indicate that the T15 monoclonal antibody and serum from immunized young adult mice which have abundant T15 antibodies are highly protective. However, non-T15 monoclonal antibodies and serum from immunized aged mice, while having high affinity for *S. pneumoniae*, were not protective. These findings indicate that while B cells of aged mice may respond normally to an infectious agent, their antibodies may be much less protective.

We are currently attempting to determine the changes in B cell generation that underlie these aging associated alterations in repertoire generation. In order to address this issue, we have analyzed H chain V gene rearrangements as they occur in the bone marrow of aged vs young mice (Decker, Linton, & Klinman, unpublished observations). The findings have proven to be extremely provocative. H chain V regions have been probed using PCR to amplify the Ig mRNA of newly emerging bone marrow B cells in aged mice. For numerous V_H gene segments, rearrangements found in bone marrow cells of aged mice are indistinguishable from rearrangements found in bone marrow cells of young adult mice. Thus, the individual members of these various V_H gene segment families are used proportionately to their utilization in young adults as are D_H and J_H gene segments. In addition, the vast majority of V_H-D_H and D_H-J_H junction have N additions. This finding is consistent with previous indications that the repertoire of V regions of aged mice is no less diverse than that of young mice (Zharhary & Klinman, 1984).

However, when rearrangements are assessed that utilize certain V_H gene segments, in particular V_1 (the V_HS107 member that participates in anti-PC responses), the pattern of expression is vastly different in newly generated bone marrow cells of aged versus young mice. These differences can be summarized as follows: 1) The frequency of V_1 utilization as compared to other members of the same V_H gene segment family is greatly increased; 2) The increase in V_1 is almost totally accounted for by its expression in association with J_{H1}.

Normally, J_{H1} is present in less than 10% of V_H-D_H-J_H rearrangements even when rearranged in conjunction with V_1. In aged bone marrow cells over 80% of V_1 rearrangements occur with J_{H1}; 3) Among rearrangements of V_1, J_{H1} occurs in association with a relatively random assortment of D_H minigene segments rather than 50% with DFL16.1 as is the case for J_{H1} in young adults; 4) Most rearrangements of V_1 in bone marrow of aged mice have no N additions which is extremely rare for all other V_H gene segments in bone marrow cells of aged mice and even V_1 in bone marrow cells of young adult mice.

This alteration in repertoire generation in aged mice has several important implications. First, the increase in V_1 utilization with J_{H1} accounts for the increase in the expression of $T15^+$ PC responsive bone marrow cells found in aged mice. Second, the increase in J_{H1} expression with D_H gene segments other than DFL16.1 is probably responsible for the increase in anti-PC responses that are positive for $V_H S107$ but are T15 negative. A tryptophan encoded by J_{H1} is the major contact residue for the choline moiety of PC and thus J_{H1} is essential for PC binding. Thus, the increase in J_{H1} with D_H regions other than DFL16.1 could contribute considerably to the expression of anti-PC antibodies that are T15 negative. Third, because the unusual rearrangements found in the bone marrow cells of aged mice are highly selective with respect to V_H gene segment utilization, it is likely that a small subset of the repertoire of aged mice is generated by a novel mechanism unlike that responsible for repertoire generation in the bone marrow of young adults or in the fetal or neonatal liver and spleen.

Although this unusual repertoire expression associated with aging had not been described previously, we have now found that it is not unique to aging. Indeed, this unusual mechanism of repertoire generation may normally be prevalent during the first 2 weeks of repertoire development in the bone marrow (as opposed to the perinatal liver and spleen). Thus, it would appear that this mechanism of repertoire expression, which is highly selective for certain V_H gene segments, may play a role in early repertoire expression but may be present only at low levels in adulthood. In aged individuals, this mechanism again becomes prevalent with the consequence that some of the resultant clonotypes may be deleterious with respect to responses to infectious agents and perhaps autoimmunity.

Clues to the Pathophysiology of Aging Associated B Cell Dysfunction

Although these findings are fascinating with respect to aging associated molecular alteration in the immune system and how they may relate to increased susceptibility to infectious disease, do they have any relevance with regard to developing strategies to ameliorate or delay dysfunction associated with aging? It should first be stated that equivalent analyses of the immune system of aged humans have not yet been carried out. Additionally, although the phenotype of altered repertoire expression in mice has been clearly established, the underlying molecular, cellular, and pathophysiologic etiology remained a mystery. This is particularly the case since any underlying causative agent would have to impact at the level of stem cell differentiation since the effects are at the earliest stages of B cell differentiation.

Recently, an important clue to the origination of altered B cell repertoire expression may have been uncovered. Several investigators have observed that erythrocyte half-life is significantly decreased in aged individuals of numerous species including mouse and man (Glass et al., 1983; Shapiro et al., 1993). In general, this foreshortened erythrocyte half life is compensated by an increase in erythropoeisis as evidenced by an increase in reticulocytes (see Fig. 4.5). The basis of the reduced erythrocyte longevity appears to be established in the bone marrow since emerging erythroid cells appear "damaged" (Shapiro et al., 1993). Since erythroid and lymphoid cells are likely to derive from a common multipotential stem cell, the possibility exists that this phenomenon could be connected to the altered B cell repertoire generation occurring in the earliest differentiated B cell progenitors. In order to test

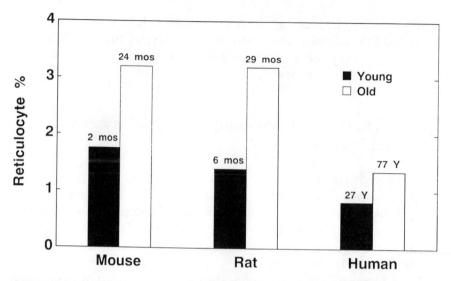

FIGURE 4.5   The percentage of reticulocytes in the blood of young and aged mice, rats and humans. (Abstracted from Magnani et al., 1988; Glass et al., 1983 and 1985.)

whether a chronic increase in erythropoeisis could affect B cell repertoire generation, we bled and iron-supplemented young mice for two weeks. Preliminary findings indicate that after such treatment the expression of the "aged" B cell repertoire phenotype could be detected. If, indeed, the altered repertoire expression of aged mice is related to decreased erythrocyte half life and increased erythropoeisis, several approaches to delay the onset of this immune dysfunction could be attempted. Additionally, the possibility that the novel B cell clonotypes generated in aged individuals may themselves damage newly generating erythrocytes should be explored.

REFERENCES

Allison, A. C., and N. E. Byars. 1992. Immunological adjuvants. *Adv. Exptl. Med. & Biol.* 327: 133.

Alt, F. W., G. D. Yancopoulos, T. K. Blackwell, C. Wood, E. Thomas,

M. Boss, R. Coffman, N. Rosenberg, S. Tonegawa, and D. Baltimore. 1984. Ordered rearrangement of immunoglobulin heavy chain variable region segments. *EMBO J. 3*: 1209.

Chandra, R. K. 1992. Effect of vitamin and trace-element supplementation on immune responses and infection in elderly subjects. *Lancet 340*: 1124.

Cillari, E., S. Milano, M. Dieli, F. Arcoleo, R. Perego, F. Leoni, G. Gromo, A. Severn, and F. Y. Liew. 1992. Thyopentin reduces the susceptibility of aged mice to cutaneous leishmaniasis by modulating CD4 T cell subsets. *Immunology 76*: 362.

Daynes, R. A., and B. A. Areneo. 1992. Prevention and reversal of some age-associated changes in immunologic responses by supplemental dehydroepiandrosterone sulfate therapy. *Aging: Immunol. & Infect. Dis. 3*: 135.

Decker, D. J., N. E. Boyle, J. Koziol, and N. R. Klinman. 1991. The expression of the immunoglobulin heavy chain repertoire in developing bone marrow B lineage cells. *J. Immunol. 146*: 350.

De Paoli, P., S. Battinstin, and G. F. Santini. 1988. Age-related changes in human lymphocyte subsets: progressive reduction of the CD4 CD45R (suppressor inducer) population. *Clin. Immunol. Immunopathol. 48*: 290.

Desiderio, S. V., G. D. Yancopoulos, M. Paskind, E. Thomas, M. Boss, N. Landau, F. W. Alt, and D. Baltimore. 1984. Insertion of N regions into heavy-chain genes is correlated with expression of terminal deoxytransferase in B cells. Nature 311: 752.

Effros, R. B., R. L. Walford, R. Weindruch, and C. Mitcheltree. 1991. Influences of dietary restriction on immunity to influenza in aged mice. *J. Gerontol. Biol. Sci. 46*: B142.

Ernst, D. N., M. V. Hobbs, B. E. Torbett, A. L. Glasebrook, M. A. Rehse, K. Bottomly, K. Hayakawa, R. R. Hardy, and W. O. Weigle. 1990. Differences in the expression profiles of CD45RB, Pgp–1, and 3G11 membrane antigens and in the patterns of lymphokine secretion by splenic CD4$^+$ T cells from young and aged mice. *J. Immunol. 145*: 1295.

Frasca, D., D. Boraschi, S. Baschieri, P. Bossu, A. Tagliabue, L. Adorini, and G. Doria. 1988. In vivo restoration of T cell functions by human IL–1 beta or its 163–171 nonapeptide in immunodepressed mice. *J. Immunol. 141*: 2651.

Feeney, A. J. 1990. Lack of N regions in fetal and neonatal mouse immunoglobulin V-D-J junctional sequences. *J. Exp. Med. 172*: 1377.

Flurkey, K., M. Stadecker, and R. A. Miller. 1992. Memory T lymphocyte hyporesponsiveness to non-cognate stimuli: a key factor in age-related immunodeficiency. *Eur. J. Immunol.* 22: 931.

Gearhart, P. J., N. Sigal, and N. R. Klinman. 1975. Heterogeneity of the BALB/c anti-phosphorylcholine antibody response at the precursor cell level. *J. Exp. Med. 141:* 56.

Glass, G. A., H. Gershon, and D. Gershon. 1983. The effect of donor and cell age on several characterisitics of rat erythrocytes. *Exp. Hematol. 11:* 987.

Glass, G. A., D. Gershon, and H. Gershon. 1985. Some characteristics of the human erythrocyte as a function of donor and cell age. *Exp. Hematol. 13:* 1122.

Goidl, E. A., J. W. Choy, J. J. Gibbons, M. E. Weksler, G. J. Thorbecke, and G. W. Siskind. 1984. Production of auto-anti-idiotypic antibody during the normal immune response. VII. Analysis of the cellular basis for the increased auto-anti-idiotype antibody production by aged mice. *J. Exp. Med. 157:* 1635.

Goidl, E. A., X. Chen, and D. H. Schulze. 1990. B cell function in the immune response of the aged. *Aging: Immunol. Infect. Dis. 2:* 135.

Grossman, A., L. Maggio-Price, J. C. Jinneman, N. S. Wolf, and P. S. Rabinovitch. 1990. The effect of long-term caloric restriction on function of T cell subsets in old mice. *Cell. Immunol. 131:* 191

Grossman, A., L. Maggio-Price, J. C. Jinneman, and P. S. Rabinovitch. 1991. Influence of aging on intracellular free calcium and proliferation of mouse T cell subsets from various lymphoid organs. *Cell. Immunol. 135:* 118.

Hallgren, H. M., N. Bergh, K. J. Rodysill, and J. J. O'Leary. 1988. Lymphocyte proliferative response to PHA and anti-CD3/Ti monoclonal antibodies, T cell surface marker expression, and serum IL–2 receptor levels as biomarkers of age and health. *Mech. Ageing Dev. 43:* 175.

Klinman, N.R. 1981. Antibody-specific immunoregulation and the immunodeficiency of aging. *J. Exp. Med. 154:* 547.

Klinman, N. R., and M. R. Stone. 1983. The role of variable region gene expression and environmental selection in determining the anti-phosphorylcholine B cell repertoire. *J. Exp. Med. 158:* 1948.

Lieberman, R., M. Potter, W. Mushinski, W. Humphrey, Jr., and S. Rudikoff. 1974. Genetics of a new IgV_H (T15 idiotype) marker in the mouse regulating natural antibody to phosphorylcholine. *J. Exp. Med. 139*: 983.

Linton, P.-J., D. J. Decker, and N. R. Klinman. 1989. Primary antibody forming cells and secondary B cells are generated from separate precursor cell subpopulations. *Cell 59*: 1049.

Linton, P.-J., D. Lo, L. Lai, G. J. Thorbecke, and N. R. Klinman. 1992. Among naive precursor subpopulations only progenitors of memory B cells originate germinal centers. *Eur. J. Immunol. 22*: 1293.

Linton, P.-J. 1993. Tolerance induction of newly generated memory B cells from aged mice. *Aging: Immunol. & Infect. Dis. 4*: 35.

Lerner, A., T. Yamada, and R. A. Miller. 1989. PGP–1[hi] T lymphocytes accumulate with age in mice and respond poorly to concanavalin A. *Eur. J. Immunol. 19*: 977.

Magnani, M., L. Rossi, V. Stocchi, L. Cucchiarini, G. Piacentini, and G. Fornaini. 1988. Effect of age on some properties of mice erythrocytes. In: *Mech. Aging and Devl. 42*: 37, Elsevier Scientific Publishers Ireland Ltd.

Nicoletti, C., C. Borghesi-Nicoleti, X. Yang, D. Schulze, and J. Cerny. 1991. Repertoire diversity of antibody response to bacterial antigens in aged mice. II. Phosphorylcholine-antibody in young and aged mice differ in both V_H/V_L gene repertoire in specificity. *J. Immunol. 147*: 2750.

Nicoletti, C., X. Yang, and J. Cerny. 1993. Repertoire diversity of antibody response to bacterial antigens in aged mice. III. Phosphorylcholine antibody from young and aged mice differ in structure and protective activity against infection with *Streptococcus pneumoniae*. *J. Immunol. 150*: 543.

Perkins, E. H., J. M. Massucci, and P. L. Glover. 1982. Antigen presentation by peritoneal macrophages from young adult and old mice. *Cell. Immunol. 70*: 1.

Perlmutter, R. M., S. T. Crews, R. Douglas, G. Sorensen, N. Johnson, N. Nivera, P. J. Gearhart, and L. Hood. 1984. The generation of diversity in phosphorylcholine-binding antibodies. *Adv. Immunol. 35*: 1.

Pierce, S. K., and N. R. Klinman. 1977. Antibody specific immunoregulation. *J. Exp. Med. 146*: 509.

Rabinowe, S. L., R. C. Nayak, K. Krisch, K. L. George, and G. S. Eisenbarth. 1987. Aging in man: Linear increase of a novel T cell subset defined by antiganglioside monoclonal antibody 3G5. *J. Exp. Med. 165*: 1436.

Riley, S. C., B. G. Froscher, P.-J. Linton, D. Zharhary, K. Marcu, and N. R. Klinman. 1989. Altered V_H gene segment utilization in the response to phosphorylcholine of aged mice. *J. Immunol. 143*: 3798.

Rodkey, L.S. 1974. Studies of idiotypic antibodies. Production and characterization of auto-anti-idiotypic antisera. *J. Exp. Med. 139*: 712.

Shapiro, S., T. Pilar, and H. Gershon. 1993. Exposure to complement-bearing immune complexes enhances the *in vitro* sequestration of erythrocytes from young but not elderly donors. *Clin. Exp. Immunol. Vol. 91* (In press).

Szakal, A. K., J. K. Taylor, J. P. Smith, M. H. Kosco, G. F. Burton, and J. G. Tew. 1988. Morphometry and kinetics of antigen transport and developing antigen-retaining reticulum of follicular dendritic cells in lymph nodes of aging immune mice. *Aging: Immunol. & Infect. Dis. 1*: 7.

Teale, J. M., and C. A. Medina. 1992. Comparative expression of adult and fetal V gene repertoire. *Intl. Rev. Immunol. 8*: 95.

Thoman, M. L., and W. O. Weigle. 1985. Reconstitution of in vivo cell-mediated lympholysis responses in aged mice with Interleukin 2. *J. Immunol. 134*: 949.

Zharhary, D., and N. R. Klinman. 1983. Antigen responsiveness of the mature and generative B cell population of aged mice. *J. Exp. Med. 157*: 1300.

Zharhary, D., and N. R. Klinman. 1984. B cell repertoire diversity to PR8-influenza virus does not decrease with age. *J. Immunol. 133*: 2285.

Zharhary, D., and N. R. Klinman. 1986a. The frequency and fine specificity of B cells responsive to 4-hydroxy–3-nitrophenyl acetyl (NP) in aged mice. *Cell Immunol. 100*: 452.

Zharhary, D., and N. R. Klinman. 1986b. A selective increase in the generation of phosphorylcholine specific B cells associated with aging. *J. Immunol. 136*: 368.

Delaying Progression of Heart Failure in the Elderly

5

Edmund H. Sonnenblick,
Thierry H. Lejemtel, and
Piero Anversa

Despite medical and surgical advances, congestive heart failure occurs with increasing frequency and remains a major source of morbidity and mortality, especially as the population ages. Prevention and treatment depends on understanding its pathophysiology and the effects of aging.

Heart failure develops with time with two components. The first is *myocardium dysfunction* due to an inadequate adaptive response to a work overload created either by primary damage or excess load, or loss of myocardium (acute myocardial infarction). Either situation leads to reactive hypertrophy of remaining cardiac cells with initial restoration of ventricular function. However, hypertrophy ultimately leads to a cascade of events that creates limited ventricular filling *(diastolic dysfunction)* and ultimately a decrease in ventricular emptying *(systolic dysfunction)*. With time, myocytes continue to be lost and hypertrophy becomes limited. Ventricular dilatation occurs as a compensation for reduced myocardial performance and a further downhill cascade occurs with mitral insufficiency, progressive wall thinning and enhanced loads on an already damaged myocardium. Thus, the initial *ventricular remodellinci*, which compromises myocardial hypertrophy and dilatation, produces a progression of ventricular dysfunction. With pump dysfunction, neurohumoral responses are activated including enhanced sympathetic tone and increased renin angiotensin activity which lead to an altered peripheral circulation and peripheral edema. The second component is *congestive heart failure*, resulting from reduced ventricular function with limited organ function, reduced exercise performance and sodium accumulation with edema. This is worsened by neurohumoral activation.

Aging, *per se*, alters structure of the heart and contributes to primary cardiac dysfunction. With aging, approximately 0.5% of cardiac myocytes are lost per year. This loss of cells is accompanied by focal fibrosis and reactive hypertrophy of the remaining myocardial cells. Thus, any other pathology is superimposed on this primary loss of cells. Hyperplasia of myocytes can also be demonstrated. With aging, contractile abnormalities occur mimicing those seen with myocardial hypertrophy. Contraction is slowed and prolonged with maintained force but with delayed relaxation. Hypertrophy of hypertension accentuates these changes. Altered relaxation may produce diastolic dysfunction well before systolic dysfunction is observed. Such contractile abnormalities are associated with changes in the delivery of calcium to the myocardium as well as the synthesis of slower contractile proteins.

To prevent progression of cardiac dysfunction and failure in the elderly, the cause of further myocyte loss must be identified and the process prevented. Adequate treatment of ischemia, salvage of myocardium with acute infarction and control of hypertension are central. Angiotensin converting enzyme inhibitors have been shown to prevent progression of mild cardiac dysfunction and to treat the symptoms related with severe cardiac dysfunction in both the younger and older patients (**SOLVD** and **SAVE** Trials).

The incidence of heart failure has increased progressively over the past three decades and it now comprises a major

source of morbidity and mortality in the American population, especially as the population ages (McKee, Castelli,
McNamara, & Kannel, 1971; Smith, 1985). Indeed, in patients
over the age of 65, heart failure has now become the most
common diagnostic related group category (DRG) for hospi-
talized patients. Thus, it not only serves as a major cause of
death and disability, but a major factor in the increasing cost
of medical care (Kannel, 1989). This increase in the incidence
of heart failure has occurred despite major advances in the
treatment of what has been thought to be primary etiological
factors initiating the problem, namely hypertension, valvular
disease, and ischemic heart disease.

For the present discussion, the primary focus is on prevention of the development and progression of heart failure. For
this, a basic model of heart failure is needed (Fig. 5.1). In general, heart failure evolves from an initial myocardial overload.
This overload might take the form of either increased pressure or volume, or loss of myocytes. In response to this overload, myocytes hypertrophy more or less to normalize the ten-
sion in the ventricular wall necessary to sustain the pressure
(Sonnenblick, Strobeck, Capasso, & Factor, 1983). Reactive hypertrophy also occurs in response to loss of myocytes, which
may be segmental as occurs with acute myocardial infarction
(Olivetti, Capasso, Meggs, Sonnenblick, & Anversa, 1991), or
diffuse as occurs in cardiomyopathies where individual or
small groups of myocytes are lost with resultant focal
fibrosis.

The response of the ventricle to the initial overload has
been termed "I'ventricular remodelling." This includes
myocyte hypertrophy, elongation, and increased ventricular
volume as well as altered ventricular shape. Following an
acute myocardial infarction, remaining viable myocardium
hypertrophies (Olivetti et al., 1991) approximately in proportion to the amount of myocytes that has been lost, so that the
mass to volume ratio of the ventricle is preserved. Aging, *per
se*, will also lead to diffuse myocyte loss and the same reactive hypertrophy as is seen with other types of overload. Hypertrophy itself then leads to alterations in mechanical behav-

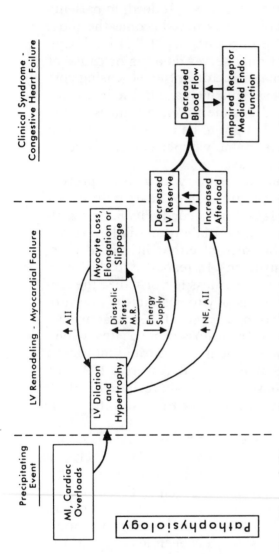

FIGURE 5.1 Heart failure evolves in three phases from the initial event where initial myocardial damage or overloading occurs through ventricular remodelling which occurs in response to the overload or damage in terms of myocardial hypertrophy and elongation. These two phases of damage and response often occur asymptomatically and one may see ventricular function declining significantly without development of significant exercise limitation or other symptoms. During the period of ventricular remodelling the neurohumoral systems may become activated with an increase in sympathetic nervous system activity and augmented activity and the renin angiotensin system. Congestive heart failure occurs as the third and final stage and is characterized by central congestion of the lungs that is generally associated with shortness of breath during exercise and eventually even at rest, as well as salt and water accumulation that produces peripheral edema and adds to central congestion. Limitations to dilation of peripheral arterioles ultimately occurs with further limitation of exercise performance. Metabolic dilatation. (Adapted from LeJemtel T.H. and Sonnenblich E.H. *Heart Failure* 9:5–7, 1993.)

ior of the myocardium with a decrease in the rate and prolongation of myocardial contraction, accompanied by a delay in relaxation. (Capasso, Malhotra, Remily, Scheyer, & Sonnenblick, 1983). This slowed contraction, however, may still produce normal force and extent of shortening due to the prolonged duration of contraction.

Reactive hypertrophy may produce some of the early manifestations of ventricular failure, i.e., *diastolic dysfunction* (Bijou, LeJemtel, & Sonnenblick, 1993; Sonnenblick, Yellin, & LeJemtel, 1983). As relaxation of cardiac muscle becomes slowed, diastolic ventricular relaxation may be impaired and result in abnormal ventricular filling. With a tachycardia, duration of diastole is further reduced. In addition, increased ventricular wall thickness, and perhaps fibrosis, which require a higher distending pressure to produce the same diastolic volume, also increase diastolic filling pressure. The development of atrial fibrillation not only may increase heart rate but produces the loss of atrial contribution to ventricular filling. Together with an unexpected salt overload, significant elevations of pulmonary pressures may occur with resultant pulmonary edema. This can occur while systolic ventricular function is well maintained and the ejection fraction is not depressed. In terms of therapeutic approaches, diastolic ventricular dysfunction requires removal of a salt overload and prolongation of diastolic time by slowing ventricular rate. Ventricular contractility (systolic function) as measured by capacity of the ventricular to empty is not reduced and thus stimulants of ventricular contractility are not needed and may even be harmful (Sonnenblick et al., 1988). Diastolic dysfunction has been documented in as much as a third of the patients who develop acute pulmonary edema in their elderly years.

With progression of myocyte loss, hypertrophy alone may not be adequate to restore myocardial mass and ventricular dilation occurs. Although stroke volume may be reasonably well maintained, an increase in diastolic volume results in a fall in ejection fraction. This describes the onset of systolic ventricular failure which correlates best with overall survival

(Kannel, 1989). As systolic dysfunction evolves, diastolic dysfunction may well persist and exacerbate hemodynamic abnormalities. Indeed, impaired systolic emptying is magnified by inadequate left ventricular filling. Of significance, decrements in ventricular performance associated with ventricular remodelling commonly occur with no overt clinical symptoms. Indeed, unless diastolic dysfunction becomes symptomatic, the fall in systolic function is generally not recognized until major depression of systolic function has already occurred. Thus, even when mild symptoms of cardiac dysfunction appear, systolic function is already markedly depressed (Bijou et al., 1993). The symptoms initially associated with the syndrome of congestive heart failure are exertion-related and mostly due to an inadequate cardiac output response and to left ventricular filling pressure. Later on, as the process progresses, symptoms become noticeable even at rest and are related to peripheral organ dysfunction along with fluid accumulation and edema (Mancini, LeJemtel, Factor, & Sonnenblick, 1986).

As the capacity of the left ventricle to empty becomes limited, elevations of diastolic ventricular filling pressure occur which may produce shortness of breath on lying down as well as with effort. Neurohumoral systems including the sympathetic nervous system and the renin angiotensin system are further activated during this time period. Sodium accumulation occurs through a number of mechanisms including increased aldosterone secretion and renal vasoconstriction. With the limitation of cardiac output, peripheral organ function is reduced producing the clinical picture of congestive heart failure. For reasons as yet undefined, as the syndrome of congestive heart failure progresses in time, metabolic dilation in muscle arterioles becomes fixed and exercise capacity is substantially reduced (Mancini et al., 1986).

Mortality from heart failure is substantial, approximating 30% to 40% in 5 years in patients who are only modestly symptomatic and as high as 50% at 1 year in patients who are symptomatic at rest (Smith, 1985). This mortality is more highly correlated with the severity of left ventricular dysfunction in terms of the ejection fraction and to a lesser extent with symptoms of congestive heart failure (Cody, 1992; Kannel, 1989).

The primary etiology of heart failure in the elderly remains the same as that for individuals of younger years (Cody, 1992). However, the problem is compounded by the process of aging itself and its impact on the myocardium, as will be dealt with more fully below. Moreover, the passage of years allows primary abnormalities such as coronary atherosclerosis to play a progressively increasing role in the evolution of the disease.

Atherosclerosis with obstructive coronary artery disease can produce heart failure through a number of mechanisms. With partial coronary occlusion, myocardial contractility may be markedly reduced even in the absence of myocardial necrosis. If coronary narrowing is partial, periods of increased oxygen demand may lead to reversible temporary ischemia with both chest pain and regional loss of myocardial contraction ("stunning") with temporary ventricular dysfunction that may be highly symptomatic. More diffuse and extensive partial obstruction of coronary arteries may reduce coronary blood flow persistently leading to decreased myocardial contraction and overall ventricular failure, although the myocardium remains viable. This latter condition, which has been termed "hibernating" myocardium, is potentially reversible with restoration of coronary blood flow. With complete obstruction of a coronary artery, generally due to thrombosis superimposed on an atherosclerotic lesion, necrosis of myocardium occurs with ventricular remodelling (Olivetti et al., 1991) and decreased ventricular function evolves depending on the size of the resultant infarction.

Hypertension commonly precedes left ventricular dysfunction in the elderly, as will be discussed below. It is also clear that when hypertension is present with diabetes, both insulin and noninsulin dependent, major myocardial dysfunction and damage are frequently present and heart failure commonly evolves from this combination (Fein & Sonnenblick, 1985). Valvular disease in the elderly provides an additional overload for the myocardium that may evolve to ventricular dysfunction. Thickening of the aortic valve is a common result of aging and fusion of the valve may lead to significant aortic stenosis (Sell & Scully, 1965) that may serve as a threat to life as well as an etiological basis for heart failure. Mitral insufficiency may also evolve from the aging of the valve with subsequent scarring and insufficiency, especially when there has been prior prolapse of the mitral valve. The aging heart itself demonstrates alterations in myocyte function and survival (Lakata, 1990), which also impact importantly on the evolution of heart disease. This, too, will be discussed more fully below.

With aging, ventricular function is altered (Gerstenblith, Lakata, & Weisfeldt, 1976; Rodeheffer et al., 1984). Cardiac output at rest, corrected for a decline as lean body mass, tends to be maintained. However, the maximum increase in cardiac output obtained with exercise declines significantly and this is associated with a decrease in the maximal oxygen consumption of the body. For the same amount of exercise, heart rate increments in the elderly are less (Stratton et al., 1992) and increased cardiac output depends on an increased diastolic volume (Rodeheffer et al., 1984). In terms of ventricular function, the rate of ventricular filling tends to decrease which may be accompanied by modest or even moderate increases in left ventricular filling pressures. Impaired left ventricular filling which occurs in the absence of decrements in systolic emptying of the heart comprises early evidence of diastolic ventricular function (Sonnenblick et al., 1988). Concommitantly, the decrease in cardiac output and stroke volume—as indicated by the ejection fraction, i.e., the ratio stroke volume to end diastolic volume—tends to decrease with age (Rodeheffer et al., 1984). By themselves, these alterations do not define heart failure but they do give some indication of ventricular dysfunction limitation of cardiovascular reserve upon which other pathological processes are imposed (Bijou et al., 1993).

Underlying these alterations in ventricular function are changes in ventricular muscle mechanics and structure. In rats, using isolated segments of cardiac myocardium, it has been demonstrated that with the process of aging, there is a progressive decrease in the velocity of myocardial contraction, a prolongation of contraction, and a delay in relaxation (Capasso et al., 1983). These alterations are accompanied by a prolongation of the electrical signal for activation (Stratton et al., 1992) and a slowing of the removal of activating calcium during relaxation (Lakata, 1990). A shift in the composition of the contractile protein myosin from a rapidly acting myosin ATPase (V,) to a slower form V3 also occurs and correlates with a reduced contractile velocity (Capasso, Malhotra, Scheyer, & Sonnenblick, 1986). Note that when experimental hypertension is superimposed on the process of aging, these changes are accelerated and amplified. Indeed, the effects of hypertrophy and aging appear additive. Of great importance in both animals (Anversa et al., 1986; Anversa, Palackal, Sonnenblick et al., 1990) and man (Olivetti, Melissari, Capasso, & Anversa, 1991) is the fact that a progressive loss of cardiac myocytes also occurs with aging. In some species of rats, in fact, this myocyte loss may be quite accelerated so that in the very elderly rat, a pathological picture consistent with a dilated cardiomyopathy develops (Anversa, Palackal, Sonnenblick et al., 1990). At this stage, ventricular performance is markedly depressed (Capasso, Palackal, Olivetti, & Anversa, 1990). This process is also accelerated by concomitant hypertension (Anversa, Palackal, Sonnenblick, Olivetti, & Capasso, 1990). In the aged rat, in addition to severe myocyte loss, reactive hypertrophy and replacement fibrosis, myocyte hyperplasia becomes evident as well (Anversao, Palackal, Sonnenblick, Olivetti, & Capasso, 1990; Anversa, Fitzpatrick, Argani, & Capasso, 1991). Whether the hypertrophy itself makes myocytes more likely to die is unknown and the basis of this myocyte loss with age remains an important subject for study and future therapy.

In normal man, 0.5% of left ventricular myocytes are lost per year (Olivetti, Melissari et al., 1991). The same loss but to a lesser extent occurs in the right ventricle. As myocytes are lost, the remaining myocytes enlarge, i.e., hypertrophy, and the lost myocytes are replaced by diffuse fibrosis. Thus, in man, the aging myocardium demonstrates reactive myocyte hypertrophy with fibrosis and ultimately may resemble a cardiomyopathy pathologically. The hypertrophy of myocytes may occur *without* an increase in overall ventricular weight and the hypertrophic state is defined by an enlargement of the myocytes themselves (Olivetti, Melissari et al., 1991). Given these hypertrophic alterations, the mechanical alterations that result are those of hypertrophy itself, whether the hypertrophy had occurred from hypertension or from the normal progressive loss of cells that occurs with aging. Any additional pathology in man is thus superimposed on this age-related loss of cells and provides some reason for the severe impact of added events such as an acute myocardial infarction in the elderly. Whether myocyte loss can be prevented or attenuated remains an interesting experimental and potentially therapeutic challenge. If this is possible it could serve as one method to prevent the progression of heart disease with aging.

In order to prevent the progression of heart failure in the elderly, primary etiologic factors require treatment whenever possible. Significant hypertension in the elderly requires control, not only to prevent strokes but to reduce the load the myocardium is required to bear (Lund-Johansen, 1988; Niarchos & Laragh, 1980; Staessen, Van Hoof, & Amory, 1988). It is very likely that treatment of hypertension is even more important in the patient who has overt or mild diabetes. In these patients, severe heart failure is common but whether early and vigorous blood pressure control can prevent this process is unknown. Also unknown is whether more vigorous control of blood sugar in diabetics will moderate progression of heart failure. In general, agents that are used to treat heart failure, as noted below, are also a value in treating the hypertension (Staessen et al., 1988), should it be an accompanying factor.

Ischemic heart disease can now be well controlled in terms of both the symptoms and the mechanical consequences of overt ischemia (Braunwald & Sobel, 1992). This requires evaluation as to the extent and severity of the ischemia, the threat to the patient in terms of specific coronary anatomy and the anticipated long-term results obtained from either medical or surgical intervention. Control of blood lipids so as to reduce the progression of atherosclerosis in the elderly remains a controversial issue. Primary prevention in this regard even in the younger individual has not proven significantly beneficial in terms of mortality, although secondary prevention has been effective to some degree.

Limitation of the extent of myocardial infarction is becoming increasingly possible through the use of thrombolysis so as to allow reperfusion and salvage of the ischemic myocardium early in the process of infarction (Braunwald & Sobel, 1992). In general, thrombolysis with reperfusion has reduced mortality following acute myocardial infarction by a third. The larger the potential infarct, the greater the benefit. Indeed, thrombolysis for myocardial infarction appears to have its greatest relative benefit in the elderly and should not be withheld for reasons of age alone. Since the extent of ventricular remodelling depends on myocardial infarct size as well, salvaging myocardium should reduce the incidence and evolution of heart failure in the elderly.

Heart failure can be considered in terms of three phases: (1) initiating events which are dealt with above, (2) ventricular remodelling which is a response to the initial damage, and (3) the endstage of congestive heart failure. Recent attention has been given to the phase of ventricular remodelling. In this phase of the evolution of heart failure, one seeks to modulate or stabilize ventricular dilatation and progressive hypertrophy so as to prevent the end-stages of the disease (Braunwald & Sobel, 1992; The SOLVD Investigators, 1991). Relative to current therapeutic modalities, angiotensin converting enzyme inhibitors have been the most effective agents (Pfeffer & SAVE Investigators, 1992; The SOLVD Investigators, 1991, 1992). The renin-angiotensin system becomes activated when cardiac function is reduced and this system greatly affects function and structure of the circulation. Space does not allow a complete description of the renin-angiotensin system but when the system becomes activated, angiotensin II leads to peripheral arteriolar vasoconstriction, release of aldosterone by the adrenals, and direct stimulation of hypertrophy of the heart and peripheral vasculature smooth muscle. Angiotensin converting enzyme (ACE) inhibitors prevent the conversion of angiotensin-I which is inactive to its active form, angiotensin-II, and thus inhibits these activities. The same converting enzyme inactivates bradykinin so that ACE inhibition leaves a greater amount of this endogenous vasodilator intact and active. In patients with mild or moderate heart failure, enalapril, which is an ACE inhibitor, has been shown to reduce morbidity as well as mortality (The SOLVD Investigators, 1991). Patients were only studied up to the age of 75 but the benefits were shown with an average age of 60. Similar benefits have been shown with other ACE inhibitors including captopril. In asymptomatic patients with decreased ejection fractions, ACE inhibitors have been shown to reduce morbidity and delay the need for hospitalization (The SOLVD Investigators, 1992).

Following a large acute myocardial infarction, ventricular dilation occurs and ACE inhibitors may be quite useful in limiting some of the consequences of the infarction. Indeed, in the SAVE (Pfeffer & SAVE Investigators, 1992) trial, captopril reduced mortality substantially as well as the development of recurrent myocardial infarction. From current data it appears that beta blockers are of the greatest benefit in reducing mortality following myocardial infarction in the first year, and that after this period, ACE inhibitors may be of great benefit in reducing further mortality as well as reinfarction (Yusuf et al., 1992).

In terms of overall protection of the heart and circulation in the elderly, one seeks to prevent atherosclerosis with its consequences of ischemia and myocyte cell loss which ultimately lead to ventricular dysfunction and failure. Whether it is possible to prevent myocyte cell loss resulting from aging alone is unclear and remains one of the great challenges for future research.

Cardiovascular function is clearly better maintained in terms of the peripheral circulation when exercise in an orderly and progressive fashion is undertaken (Mancini et al., 1986). This leads to an improvement in peripheral circulatory responses and a sense of improved well-being. Clearly, exercise improves the quality of life. Prolongation of life will still remain to a large extent in the realm of myocyte survival.

REFERENCES

Anversa P, Fitzpatrick D, Argani S, & Capasso JM: Myocyte nutotic division in the aging mammalian rat heart. *Circ Res 69*:1159–1164, 1991.

Anversa P, Hiler B, Ricci R, et al.: Myocyte cell loss and myocyte hypertrophy in the aging rat. *J Am Coll Cardiol 8*:1441–1448, 1986.

Anversa P, Palackal T, Sonnenblick EH, et al.: Myocyte cell loss and myocyte cellular hyperplasia in the hypertrophied aging rat heart. *Circ Res 67*:871–885, 1990.

Anversa P, Palackal T, Sonnenblick EH, Olivetti G, & Capasso JM: Hypertensive cardiomyopathy: Myocyte hyperplasia in mammalian rat heart. *J Clin Invest 85*:994–997, 1990.

Bijou R, LeJemtel, TH, & Sonnenblick EH: From left ventricular dysfunction to heart failure in the elderly patient. *Am J Geriatric Cardiol 2*:14–25, 1993.

Braunwald E, & Sobel BE: Coronary blood f low and myocardial ischemia. In *Heart Disease*, ed. E. Braunwald. W.B. Saunders, Phila. pp 1161–1199, 1991.

Capasso JM, Malhotra A, Remily RM, Scheuer J, & Sonnenblick EH: Effects of age on mechanical and electrical performance of rat myocardium. *Am J Physiol 245*:H72-H81, 1983.

Capasso JM, Malhotra A, Scheuer J, & Sonnenblick EH: Myocardial biochemical, contractile, and electrical performance after imposition of hypertension in young and old rats. *Circ Res 58*:445–460, 1986.

Capasso JM, Palackal T, Olivetti G, & Anversa P: Severe myocardial dysfunction induced by ventricular remodeling in aging rat hearts. *Am J Physiol 259*:HlO86–1096, 1990.

Cody J: Characteristics of the elderly patient with congestive heart failure. *Am J Geriatric Cardiol 1*:30–41, 1992.

Fein FS, & Sonnenblick EH: Diabetic cardiomyopathy. *Prog in Cardiovasc Dis 4*:255–270, 1985.

Gerstenblith G, Lakatta EG, & Weisfeldt ML: Age changes in myocardial function and exercise response. *Prog Cardiovasc Dis 19*:1–21, 1976.

Kannel, WB: Epidemiological aspects of heart failure. *Cardiol Clin* 7:1–9, 1989.

Lakata EG: Changes in cardiovascular function with aging. *Europ H J ll*:(Suppl C):22–29, 1990.

Lund-Johansen P: The hemodynamics of the aging cardiovascular system. *J Cardiovasc Pharm 12 (Supp 8)*:520–530, 1988.

McKee PA, Castelli WP, McNamara PM, & Kannel WB: The natural history of congestive heart failure: The Framingham Study. *N Engl J Med 285*:144–146, 1971.

Mancini D, LeJemtel TH, Factor S, & Sonnenblick EH: The central and peripheral components of heart failure. *Am J Med 8 0 (suppl 2B)*:2–13, 1986.

Niarchos AP, & Laragh JH: Hypertension in the elderly. Modern Concepts. *Cardiovas Dis 49*:43–54, 1980.

Olivetti G, Capasso JM, Meggs LG, Sonnenblick EH, & Anversa P: Cellular basis of chronic ventricular remodeling after myocardial infarction in rats. *Circ Res 68*:856–869, 1991.

Olivetti G, Melissari M, Capasso JM, & Anversa P: Cardiomyopathy of the aging human heart. Myocyte loss and reactive cellular hypertrophy. *Circ Res 68*:1560–1568, 1991.

Pfeffer MA, & SAVE Investigators: Effect of captopril on mortality and morbidity in patients with left ventricular dysfunction after myocardial infarction. *NEJM 327*:669–677, 1992.

Rodeheffer RJ, Gerstenblith G, Becker LC, Fleg JL, Weisfeldt ML, & Lakatta EG: Exercise output is maintained with advancing age in healthy human subjects; cardiac dilatation and increased stroke volume compensate for a diminished heart rate. *Circulation 69*: 203–213, 1984.

Sell S, & Scully RE: Aging, changes in the aortic and mitral valves. Histological and histochemical studies, with observation on the pathogenesis of calcific aortic stenosis and calcification of the mitral annulus. *Am J Physiol 46*: 345–365, 1965.

Smith WM: Epidemiology of congestive heart failure. *Am Cardol 55*:3A–8A, 1985.

The SOLVD Investigators: Effect of enalapril on mortality and the development of heart failure in asymptomatic patients with reduced left ventricular ejection fractions. *NEJM 327*:685–691, 1992.

The SOLVD Investigators: Effect of enalapril on survival in patients
    with reduced left ventricular ejection fractions and congestive
    heart failure. *NEJM 325*:293–302, 1991.
Sonnenblick EH, Strobeck JE, Capasso JM, & Factor SM: Ventricu-
    lar Hypertrophy: Models and methods in perspectives in car-
    diovascular research—Cardiac hypertrophy in hypertension.
    Ed: Katz AM, Tarasi RC, and Dunbbar JB. Vol 8:13–. Raven
    Press NY, 1983.
Sonnenblick EH, Yellin E, & LeJemtel TH: Congestive heart failure
    and intact systolic ventricular performance. *Heart Failure 4(4/
    5)*:164–173, 1988.
Staessen J, Gagard R, Van Hoof R, & Amory A: Antihypertensive
    drug therapy in elderly hypertensive subjects: Evidence of pro-
    tection. *J Cardiovasc Pharm 12 (Suppl 8)*:S33–38, 1988.
Stratton JR, Cerqueira MD, Schwartz RS, et al.: Differences in car-
    diovascular responses to isoproterenol in relation to age and
    exercise training in healthy men. *Circulation 86*:504–512, 1992
Yusuf S, Pepine CJ, Carces C, et al.: Effect of enalapril on myocar-
    dial infarction and unstable angina in patients with low ejec-
    tion fractions. *Lancet 340*:1173–1178, 1992.

Delay of Functional Decline in Alzheimer's Disease: An Experimental and Theoretical Perspective

6

Carl W. Cotman

INTRODUCTION

People over 65 years old are the fastest growing segment of the American population. Vitally important to the quality of life is maintenance of cognitive function. Though decline may occur, age alone need not result in the loss of such function. Both animals and human beings display a marked heterogeneity in brain physiology and cognitive performance at later ages. While some succumb to disease and deterioration, certain individuals manage to "age successfully," maintaining high levels of intellectual functionality throughout life. Discovering how some individuals live the last years of life unhindered by a debilitating cognitive handicap has the potential to extend to others the same privilege.

Age-related dementia nominally results in the loss of cognitive function, affecting, in particular, the ability to recall events. Dementia's most prevalent cause is Alzheimer's disease (AD), although vascular disease often co-exists with dementia or is itself a cause. An etiologic link to age constitutes one of the most salient features of dementia and provides a clue that any comprehensive hypothesis must take into account. AD is very rare in persons under 65 years of age, is found in approximately 12% of the 65–74 year-old population, yet rises to over 45% in the 85 + population.

The second prominent feature of the disease is its effect on the processes of molecular, cellular, and behavioral plasticity. As originally described by William James in 1890, behavioral plasticity refers to any meaningful change in behavior. AD compromises the ability to learn and recall information and the ability to control and execute meaningful changes in behavior. Early in the course of the disease, patients cannot recall names or places recently experienced. As the disease progresses, the individual develops an inability to control behavior and may display increased aggressiveness, wandering, and agitation. The ability to execute meaningful changes in behavior is lost. Ironically and tragically, the disease selectively attacks the most plastic among the brain's centers, striking first the malleable circuits engaged in learning and memory, then undermines the more stable functions responsible for higher cognition and behavioral control, finally compromising the personality itself. As a result, it is increasingly clear that AD begins its relentless destruction of the brain with subtle assaults on the brain where it is most pliant and yielding.

In this chapter, we shall present recent findings aimed at defining the mechanisms that maintain function with aging versus those participating in decline and leading to dementia. We suggest that brain plasticity helps to maintain function through various cellular and molecular mechanisms (functional plasticity), but that as function declines some of these same mechanisms are recruited into events that compromise neuronal function, disrupt neuronal circuits, and in some cases, lead to neuronal death (dysfunctional plasticity). We further suggest that one of the molecules that accumulates with aging, β-amyloid, organizes and drives dysfunction.

FUNCTIONAL VERSUS DYSFUNCTIONAL PLASTICITY

A growing body of evidence suggests that the machinery responsible for neuronal plasticity in the mammalian brain plays complex roles in both the protection and eventual collapse of cognitive function during aging and disease. Although the aged nervous system has a capacity to compensate for significant damage and stress, the ability of the brain's internal machinery to compensate for damage is not unlimited. In fact, once they pass the point of balance between plasticity and pathology, the very mechanisms that once prevented cognitive and behavioral deficits apparently serve to accelerate loss of function.

Our general hypothesis is that AD does not have a single "cause" but rather develops and progresses as a result of the accumulation of challenges, losses in regulation, and the diminished ability to compensate. Importantly, though, this accumulation appears to be not merely additive but, as each of the processes is interrelated, becomes synergistic and eventually leads to destructive molecular cascades (Fig. 6.1).

The general intellectual framework engendered by this hypothesis has important implications for a research strategy in that it demands an integrated multi-disciplinary basic science/clinical program to investigate its key questions and assumptions. Second, the hypothesis has implications both for understanding the origins of neurodegenerative disease and finding potential therapies to slow its progress. It suggests that early detection of cognitive decline and timely intervention have the greatest potential for preventing or slowing molecular cascades before they no longer can be controlled (Fig. 6.1A, dashed line). In addition, the general hypothesis suggests that plasticity processes are operative throughout aging and disease and that it should be possible to draw upon them, strengthening those still operative to increase the brain's natural resilience and resistance to deterioration (Fig. 6.1B).

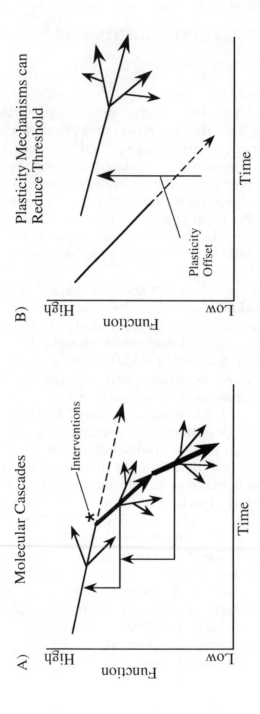

FIGURE 6.1 General mechanisms leading to brain dysfunction. A) The development of dysfunction in the aged brain appears to arise from a series of molecular and cellular events that add up to create autodestructive cascades. Identifying those events early in the cascade and finding means to regulate them will prolong high function. B) Some molecules such as β-amyloid organize and drive these cascades. As illustrated in this chapter, some plasticity mechanisms can offset loss, reduce threshold, and maintain function.

CELL LOSS STIMULATES THE REMAINING NEURONS TO REGENERATE NEW NEURAL CIRCUITRIES

With aging, and to a greater degree in AD, neurons degenerate in select areas of the brain, e.g., the entorhinal cortex, a part of the temporal lobe. Cell loss, over a period of time, causes a loss of connectivity and therefore, function. It would be surprising, however, if the brain did not have some adaptive mechanisms to compensate for specific cell loss in circuits. Whereas in some tissues cells are added by cell division, this mechanism is not known to occur in the mature and aged brain. Therefore, the remaining cells utilize other compensatory mechanisms.

In animal models it is possible to create controlled entorhinal cell loss and examine the consequences on the remaining neurons and their circuitries. After entorhinal lesions, synapses initially degenerate and function declines as a consequence of degeneration. But then over time, if the lesion spares some entorhinal neurons, the remaining ones sprout new connections and minimize functional loss (Cotman, 1990; Cotman, Gomez-Pinilla, & Kahle, 1993). We have suggested, as have others, that axon sprouting is a critical plasticity mechanism that is part of an ongoing brain maintenance program. The healthy cells make new connections and regenerate new circuits (Fig. 6.2).

Recently we developed a lesion model in the rat that allows the examination of functional changes after partial lesions of the entorhinal cortex and subsequent sprouting and synaptic reorganization of remaining perforant path fibers (Kahle, Ulas, & Cotman, 1993). The left entorhinal cortex was extensively lesioned using electrolytic lesions, whereas approximately one third of the right entorhinal cortex was lesioned. This resulted in the degeneration of a portion of medial perforant path and a robust sprouting response in the dentate gyrus molecular layer confirmed by cholinergic sprouting, while a proportion of perforant path fibers remained intact, allowing the electrophysiological and pharmacological char-

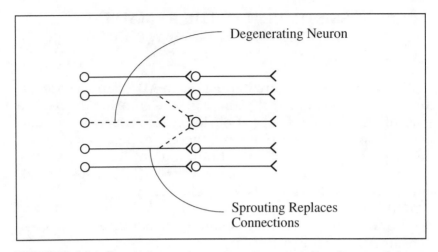

FIGURE 6.2 Sprouting can regenerate partially damaged brain circuitry. When a neuron degenerates the neighboring healthy cells form new synapses to replace those lost.

acterization of the synaptic activity in the reorganized dentate molecular layer. This approach provided data on sprouting mechanisms triggered by loss of a fraction of the cells of the entorhinal cortex.

The electrophysiological characteristics of the sprouted dentate gyrus was assessed both 2 days and 2 weeks post-lesion using an *in vitro* hippocampal slice preparation and extracellular recording (Fig. 6.3). This corresponds to the time course of lesioned-induced fiber sprouting studied previously; at 2 days post-lesion sprouting has not commenced, but by 2 weeks post-lesion fiber sprouting is robust. In unlesioned slices, medial perforant path responses were high amplitude, downward-going field potentials that exhibited depression in response to paired stimuli 40–800 ms apart (paired-pulse depression; Fig. 6.3). In contrast, medial perforant path responses recorded in 2 day post-lesion slices were low amplitude, upward-going field potentials. By 2 weeks post-lesions, medial perforant path responses recovered to relatively high amplitude, downward-going field potentials similar to that re-

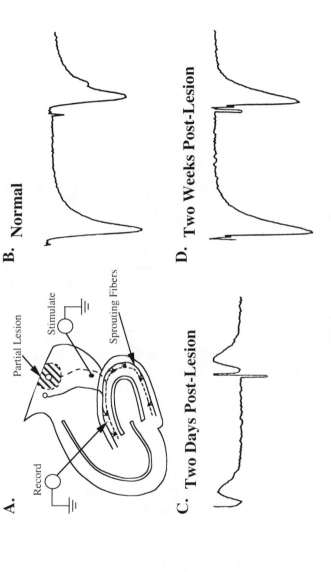

A.

Record

Partial Lesion

Stimulate

Sprouting Fibers

B. Normal

C. Two Days Post-Lesion

D. Two Weeks Post-Lesion

FIGURE 6.3 Synaptic responses recorded from the dantate gyrus molecular layer recovered in amplitude and shape two weeks after partial entorhinal lesions. Stimulating and recording electrodes were placed as in the drawing (A). CA1, CA1 pyramidal layer; CA3. The field potentials measurable 2 days post-lesion (C) were considerably smaller and of opposite polarity when compared to field potentials from unlesioned animals (B). By 2 weeks post-lesion, substantial field potentials similar to field potentials from unlesioned animals were recorded (D). Note also that unlesioned and 2 week post-lesion slices exhibited consistent paired-pulse depression, a form of synaptic plasticity similar to the control undamaged slice. Scale bars, 0.5 mV, 9 ms.

corded from unlesioned slices. Also comparable to unlesioned slices, responses recorded in 2 week post-lesion slices exhibited consistent paired-pulse depression that was virtually as robust as paired-pulse depression in unlesioned animals.

The entorhinal lesion model in rodents has allowed the identification of plasticity events that take place after cell loss. In general, such lesions result in a systematic rearrangement of the existing circuitry and the rebuilding of connections (Cotman, 1990; Cotman, 1989; Cotman et al., 1993). Like inputs take preference and replace connections by making similar connections using the same neurotransmitter, particularly after partial lesions. In addition, however, some afferent systems using different neurotransmitters also sprout. One of the more interesting and robust ones is the cholinergic input from the medial septal area (Cotman et al., 1993). This sprouting of cholinergic input may act as an additional source of acetylcholine to enhance cholinergic function. Increases in cholinergic function have been demonstrated to enhance hippocampal function in old animals both pharmacologically and via cholinergic brain transplants. Perhaps this type of heterologous sprouting serves a similar function, particularly when some outlined input is maintained. These regenerative processes operate not only in the mature brain but equally well with a slight delay in the aged brain.

In addition to restoring connectivity, sprouting probably also plays a key role in maintaining neurotrophic factor interactions between neurons. Neurotrophic factors are a class of proteins which aid in neuronal survival, differentiation and growth (see Cotman et al., 1993 for discussion). Neurons depend on these factors and largely derive them from their target neurons. It is well-established that if neurons lose their connections to their target, they degenerate primarily because they lose neurotrophic factors. For example, transection of the axon of septal neurons causes their atrophy and eventual degeneration but these neurons can be rescued if the neurotrophic factors either FGF-2 or NGF are provided before or immediately after transection. Previously, we and others have shown that after injury, there is a rise in neurotrophic factor levels (e.g., FGF–2) which initiates and stimulates regenerative growth. The increase then subsides as neurons develop an augmented set of trophic interactions. Reestablishment of trophic support is probably a key aspect of this regenerative process.

REGENERATIVE GROWTH ALSO OCCURS IN THE AD BRAIN

Sprouting may also occur in early AD. Studies in animal models predict that in the human brain similar events may occur. The variety of anatomical markers defined from animal models allows the investigation of axon sprouting in postmortem tissues collected from AD cases.

The cognitive and memory deficits in AD are tied to a functional disconnection of the ventral medial temporal lobe and association cortices. There is extensive loss and the presence of extensive pathology, particularly in layer two of the entorhinal cortex which disrupts the entorhinal hippocampal pathway. Compounding this is damage to the output of the circuit, the CA 1 subicular, and the limbic-associated cortical connections mediated by subicular projections. In this way, the hippocampus is disconnected from both input and output elements (Hyman et al., 1984, 1990). Rebuilding connections via sprouting and establishing new synapses would offset neuronal loss and maintain function longer in aging and AD. In addition to cell loss there is an associated accumulation of several unusual features in AD brains. As neurons degenerate, many of them form neurofibrillary tangles, which as originally described by Alzheimer (1907) may indicate "the site where once the neurons had been located." Further, as Alzheimer also noted, "dispersed over the cortex by large numbers, especially in the upper layers, miliary foci could be found which represented the sites of deposition of a particular substance in the cerebral cortex." These are called senile plaques. Thus neurofibrillary tangles and senile plaques are the primary pathological structures in the AD brain. Until recently, most studies on AD have focused on the study of these events and the manner in which they cause the breakdown of the elaborate circuitries in the brain.

It is clear from a variety of cellular and molecular studies that in AD, neurons have the basic molecular machinery to regenerate and indeed do regenerate connections. As predicted from animal models, there is a sprouting of cholinergic input to the hippocampus, induction of excitatory amino acid receptors, and the appearance of several molecular markers, indicative of regenerative growth (Geddes et al., 1985; Hyman et al., 1987). In AD, however, the sprouts from many of the cholinergic and other fibers appear to be associated with senile plaques, an event not predicted from animal models (Geddes et al., 1986). For example, in Figure 6.4A fibers appear to be attracted into the maturing plaque; they appear to be targeting the plaque area. In Figure 6.4B, a fiber almost does a loop turn as it enters the plaque which again suggests an abberent type growth. In fact, Ramon y Cajal also noticed this growth and commented, "It appears that the sprouts have been attracted to the region of the plaque under the influence of some special neurotrophic substance" (Cajal, 1928). In the dentate gyrus the plaques appear to contain a concentration of the bulk of cholinergic fibers in the latter stages of the disease that greatly exceeds that which is found in the surrounding neuropile. In addition to cholinergic fibers, many other fibers appear to sprout into plaques. The plaque appears to concentrate regenerative growth events, an example of dysfunctional plasticity.

The extent that neurites become engaged in the plaque environment, rather than with their normal neuronal counterparts, indicates an abberent type of sprouting reaction which is distinct from that which occurs in the young, mature, and healthy aged brain in animals or humans. Sprouting associated with this could compromise the ability to form synapses, disrupt trophic influences and place neurons at a greater risk for degeneration. Indeed the presence of neuritic pathology is a hallmark of the AD brain and is associated with a distinct form of senile plaque, indicative of a breakdown of circuitry.

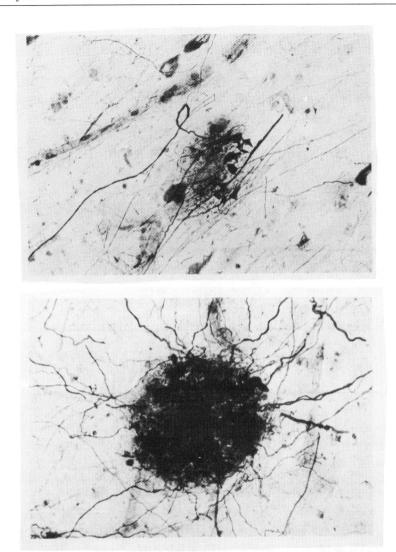

FIGURE 6.4 Neuritic plaques in the AD brain. These plaques consist of a core of β–amyloid, FGF-2 (a neurotrophic factor), heparin sulfate proteoglycan(s) (an ideal substrate for neurite growth), and other substances which stimulate neuron process growth. β-amyloid both attracts processes and promotes their degeneration. Both plaques (A and B) have attracted extensive neuritic growth. Some of the processes appear dystrophic (swollen and fragmented).

Recently, a group of investigators (McKee et al., 1991) have reported that neuritic pathology as revealed by immunoreactivity for tau protein is strongly correlated with clinically assessed dementia. This finding was evident, even in brains with few neurofibrillary tangles. In this study both dystrophic neurites and neurofibrillary tangle numbers were highly correlated with dementia rating scale scores in CA1, entorhinal cortex, superior cortex and inferior parietal cortex. It is fair to conclude that a consensus is developing, suggesting that dystrophic neurite events (including synaptic loss; Terry et al., 1991) may be a more sensitive correlate of clinical dementia than all types of plaques or neurofibrillary tangles. Neuritic abnormalities would indeed appear to be associated with a decrease in synapse number and may be part of an ongoing early atrophy process. This would further reflect the ability to successfully regulate regenerative growth and establish new connections.

It is possible that the dysfunction associated with beta amyloid (Aβ) and amyloid precursor protein (APP) is related to their normal function. Recent evidence suggests that APP has the capacity to promote neurite outgrowth and adhesion (Milward et al., 1992). In turn, we would suggest that Aβ is involved in neurite retraction under normal conditions. That is, Aβ is produced in order to reduce sprouting and connectivity. The accumulation of the substance in plaques and to a degree as fine deposits in the extracellular space with aging withdraws sprouts, prevents growth and retards turnover.

THE PRESENCE OF NEURITIC SENILE PLAQUES INDICATES DISRUPTED NEURAL CIRCUITRY

Neuritic plaques represent a key factor causing the disruption of neural circuitry. They are, in a sense, a biogenetic force which can contribute to the unraveling of neurocircuits, displacement of healthy neurons, and the siphoning of regenerative events into pathology. Accordingly, it is of interest to define the mechanisms that lead to plaque formation and

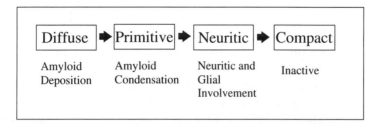

FIGURE 6.5 Stages in the biogenesis of a senile plaque. The top line illustrate the stages identified from neuropathology studies. The lower line proposes a series of molecular events which underlie plaque biogenesis.

maturation, both as a means to understand the genesis of this specific organelle and also as a means to better understand some of the forces leading to AD pathology.

Figure 6.5 summarizes the basic classic stages in plaque formation as defined by neuropathologists and proposes a new model to translate these states into molecular terms. In essence the model proposes a series of transformations whereby the major molecule contained in plaques, β-amyloid, accumulates in excess and begins a process of condensation. This is later followed by a folding of amyloid into a β-pleated sheet structure and the addition of other components. This is driven by the adhesive capacity of β-amyloid to itself, other components and time. The next stage, called the neuritic plaque, appears to be the one associated with AD. In the next stage, the plaque becomes associated with glial cells (microglia and astrocytes) and neurites begin to sprout into the developing plaque. We suggest that the neuritic plaque signals the onset of dysfunctional plasticity, associated with key deregulated molecular events. These involve both β-amyloid and select growth factors.

β-amyloid, which is derived from a large precursor protein, has long been considered to be biologically inert. Recent evidence initially from our laboratory, demonstrated that β-amyloid has growth promoting properties (Whitson et al., 1989, 1990). Ironically, however, as β-amyloid accumulates it places neurons at risk and lowers the threshold for cell death (Koh et al., 1990; Mattson et al., 1992). Soluble Aβ appears to be neurotrophic in low density tissue cultures optimized for the observation of trophic responses. These cultures display short-term survival enhancement in response to soluble Aβ 1–28 and 1–42 and a significant increase in axonal elongation in response to Aβ 1–42 (Whitson et al., 1990). When Aβ is present in an aggregated assembly state, it retains its neuritic and outgrowth promoting properties; however, the neurites in contact with Aβ aggregates exhibit dystrophic morphology similar to that seen in the environment of the neuritic plaque (Pike et al., 1992a,b). The neuritic processes appear to grow toward Aβ aggregates, but once in contact become bulbous along their length and eventually fragment. Processes of attraction and destruction represent one of the molecular paradoxes emerging in the study of AD pathology. Seemingly, growth places the processes of neurons at risk for subsequent destruction.

In addition to the trophic promoting properties of β-amyloid, the trophic environment of the plaque is further enhanced by an accumulation of various neurotrophic factors such as basic fibroblast growth factor (FGF–2). FGF–2 is a neurotrophic factor which acts on the majority of brain neurons, particularly glutamate neurons (see Cotman et al., 1993; Baird & Bohlen, 1991). For example, FGF–2 enhances the survival of cortical and hippocampal neurons and stimulates neuritic outgrowth when added to cultures of these neurons.

Recently, we and others have identified FGF–2 within senile plaques (Gomez-Pinilla et al., 1990; Stopa et al., 1990). There is an increase in the FGF–2 in the AD brain. Although the increased levels may be providing additional trophic support to neurons under stress in the AD brain, the highest concentrations appear in senile plaques. The localization of FGF–2 within pathological structures is likely involved in the stimulation of neuronal growth into the plaque thereby enhancing the contact between Aβ and neurons and placing these cells at risk.

To date we have not been able to identify FGF–2 in the precursor to neuritic plaques, the diffuse plaque. FGF–2, for example, is not present in cerebellar plaques, the canine brain, or early Down Syndrome where diffuse plaques prevail or are exclusively present. In other words, a trophic factor that could be working to restore function becomes concentrated in a microbiogenetic environment, which is associated with the progression of AD pathology. Studies on the progression of senile plaques may allow identification of new mechanisms in AD. Senile plaques per se are not the cause of the disease, but they are one of the central risk factors that contribute to neuronal dysfunction.

RECURSIVE MOLECULAR CASCADES MAY DRIVE DYSFUNCTIONAL PLASTICITY

Several molecular events in the plaque environment merge into a series of recursive cascades that drive the development of dysfunctional plasticity. Since current epidemiological data suggests that increasing age may correspond to an increased probability of the events leading to AD pathology, it seems intuitive that a set of events drives these pathological processes with an ever-increasing rate and severity over time. Given this possibility, we investigated the hypothesis that Aβ itself might stimulate cells in the plaque environment to produce more FGF–2. Indeed, exposure of primary astrocytes and microglia to Aβ 1–42 increased the amount of FGF–2 (Araujo & Cotman, 1992). Furthermore, there is evidence to support a potential role for positive feedback loops in AD pathology. FGF–2 induces a five to tenfold increase in APP mRNA (Quon, Catalano, & Cordell, 1990), and a twofold increase in NGF secretion (Yoshida & Gage, 1991). In return, both FGF–2 and NGF have been reported to increase APP production (Schubert, Jin, Saitoh, & Cole, 1989), and NGF may potentiate the toxicity of Aβ 1–40 *in vitro* (Yankner, Caceres, & Duffy, 1990).

Thus one potential molecular feedback loop might be as follows: FGF–2 stimulates an increase in APP levels, APP in turn increases the probability of Aβ production, Aβ then in-

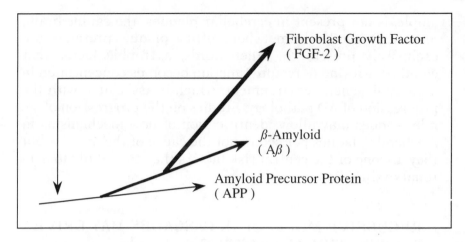

FIGURE 6.6 Example of a molecular cascade that drives senile plaque formation, attracts neurites to plaques and contributes to dysfuntional plasticity. The feedback loop of FGF-2 stimulating APP formation amplifies the biogenetic event.

creases bFGF production in the plaque environment—further stimulating APP production (Fig. 6.6). The initiation of this type of cascade illustrates how events in isolation, which might have a normal regulatory role, can enter into a destructive sequence and drive dysfunctional plasticity.

Aβ AS AN ORGANIZING AND RISK FACTOR TO NEURONS

As Aβ accumulates we have suggested that it becomes a risk factor to neurons making the cells more susceptible to insults such as low glucose, minor seizures and other toxins such as those causing oxidative injury. Because Aβ continues to accumulate in the brain, self-assembles and attracts or drives other reactions, it acts as an organizing factor for disease progression.

A potential risk factor in AD is hypoglycemia. Low cerebral glucose metabolism has been identified in aging and early AD in several studies, and proposed as a contributing factor in AD pathology and dementia (Hoyer, Oesterreich, & Wagner, 1988). This suggested that hypoglycemia could represent a risk factor for cell death when combined with Aβ. In order to evaluate this possibility, mature mouse cortical cultures were exposed to a brief period of glucose deprivation in combination with soluble Aβ 1–42. This caused severe cell loss, while control cultures exposed to glucose deprivation alone exhibit only mild damage (Copani, Koh, & Cotman, 1991). Interestingly, cell death induced by hypoglycemia is mediated by excitotoxic mechanisms *in vivo* (Wieloch, 1985) and *in vitro* (Monyer & Choi, 1988). In accordance with these data, the administration of a non-competitive NMDA receptor antagonist (MK–801) in conjunction with glucose deprivation and soluble Aβ as described above is neuroprotective (Copani et al., 1991). These results support a role for unaggregated Aβ in the initiation of neuronal damage by increasing the vulnerability of neurons to other risk factors.

Aβ DECREASES THE THRESHOLD FOR NEURONAL INJURY AND DEATH

The induction of neuritic dystrophy in the processes of neurons exposed to Aβ suggests more direct toxic effects on the cells themselves. In fact, a toxic response to Aβ peptides follows the initial period of trophic interactions observed with soluble Aβ; after several days *in vitro* Aβ 1–42 exposure results in decreased cell survival in the same low density culture system used for the assessment of trophic interactions (Pike, Walencewicz, Glabe, & Cotman, 1991a, 1991b). Aβ 1–40 exposure over several days also results in neurite retraction and cell death in hippocampal cultures (Yankner et al., 1990). The data by Yankner et al., however, suggested a direct toxic effect of Aβ. How can the same molecule have different opposing actions?

Over time Aβ collects in the aged brain as aggregates that increase in size and, as noted above, form senile plaques. For this reason we examined the possibility that the assembly state of soluble Aβ may influence its biological activity. It may be that soluble Aβ enhances neuron growth, though is a risk factor, whereas aggregated Aβ is toxic to neurons. Aβ was incubated for several days so that it aggregated and was compared to newly solublized non-aggregated Aβ. Indeed, exposure of high density immature hippocampal cultures to aggregated Aβ 1–42 causes severe cell death and degeneration. Neither soluble Aβ 1–42 nor 1–28 exhibit toxic cellular effects in this culture paradigm, although the increased neuritic outgrowth noted in low density immature hippocampal cultures in response to soluble Aβ 1–42 is apparent (Pike et al., 1991a). In a more recent study, the variety of Aβ peptide fragments examined was expanded. Of ten different Aβ peptide lengths, only peptides which formed an aggregated assembly state were toxic in the high density developing hippocampal culture system; prevention or reversal of the aggregated assembly state was effective in attenuating this toxicity (Pike et al., 1992a). Interestingly, other fragments of APP (the secreted form) can exert a protective role (Mattson et al., 1993).

Thus, Aβ appears to be a molecule which may organize and catalyze subsequent pathology, perhaps by altering the threshold of neurons to neuritic retraction, dysfunction, and degeneration. While it is clear that Aβ can initiate neuronal death and degeneration, the mechanisms by which the cells die is undefined. It is important to clarify this mechanism in order to develop interventions.

NATURAL CELL DEATH (APOPTOSIS) MAY CAUSE NEURONAL LOSS IN AGING AND AD

In general, cells die by a mechanism of necrosis or apoptosis [see Wyllie et al. for review (Wyllie, Kerr, & Currie, 1980)]. Necrosis is typically responsible for cell loss following acute external insults, e.g., head trauma and lesions. Apoptosis (sometimes also called natural cell death) occurs in response to internal metabolic cues that trigger a molecular program of cellular self-destruction. In necrosis there is a gross swelling of the mitochondria, rupture of nuclear, organelle, and plasma membranes, and a corresponding dissolution of lysosomes and ribosomes. In contrast, apoptosis is characterized by condensation of the nucleus, cytoplasm, and chromatin, and the formation of cell-surface protrusions termed blebs. In this way cells undergoing apoptosis maintain the integrity of their membranes until quite late in the degenerative process. An additional mechanism in the apoptotic pathway is the activation of endogenous endonucleases resulting in DNA fragmentation, thereby destroying a residual genetic message.

Recently we have described a series of morphologic and biochemical changes characteristic of apoptosis in cultured neurons exposed to Aβ. Figure 6.7, for example, shows a scanning electron micrograph of Aβ-induced membrane blebbing. These cells exhibit a variety of ultrastructural phenomena characteristic of apoptosis including shrinking, membrane blebbing, chromatin condensation, the maintenance of intact organelles, and the presence of isolated pycnotic nuclei. Furthermore, these cells exhibited a classic apoptotic pattern of DNA fragmentation (Loo et al., 1993). These findings suggest that apoptosis may be a significant mechanism of neuronal loss in AD and possibly aging.

The hypothesis that apoptosis could contribute to AD is attractive for a variety of reasons. In contrast to the simultaneous loss of groups of neurons typical of lesion-induced necrosis, the prolonged and progressive loss of isolated neurons in AD pathology is consistent with an apoptotic mechanism of cell death. Similarly, the identification of a relationship between some toxins and apoptosis suggests that environmental risk factors may contribute to the induction of cell death in some instances. For example, dioxin activates an apoptotic pathway in thymocytes (Orrenius, McConkey, Bellomo, & Nicotera, 1989). More closely related to the case of neurodegenerative disease, 1-methyl–4-phenylpyridinium (MPP+), a toxin which causes Parkinson's-type pathology in rats, monkeys and humans, also produces changes characteristic of

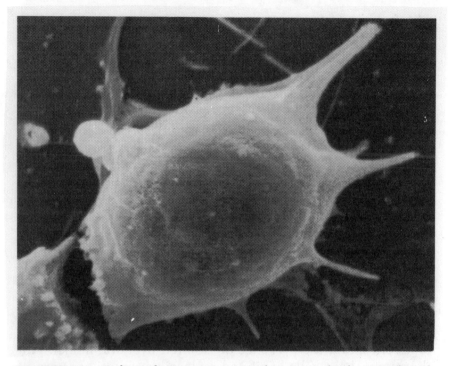

FIGURE 6.7 Cultured neurons exposed to β-amyloid are induced
to initiate an internal program that actively causes their death. This
form of natural cell death (apoptosis is proposed to contribute to
cell loss in aging and age-related neurodegenerative disorders. One
of the hallmarks of apoptosis is the formation of extensive surface
protrusion called blebs. A) scanning electron micrograph of a
normal neuron, B) scanning electron micrograph of neuron treated
with β-amyloid and showing extensive blebbing. (*Source*: Loo et al.,
1993.)

apoptosis in cerebellar granule cell cultures (Dipasquale,
Marini, & Youle, 1991).

In fact, it may be that the controlled removal of neurons which
have become dystrophic and dysfunctional could be an adaptive
mechanism in AD, and that an apoptotic pathway may be initiated in an attempt to retain function in a disintegrating neuronal
circuitry without damaging the connections of nearby but unaf-

fected neurons. Cell death appears to continue unabated. β-amyloid may be serving as one signal which fails to turn off and ultimately destroys cells needlessly by natural mechanisms (Cotman & Anderson, 1993). At present, however, definitive evidence that apoptosis contributes to neuronal death *in vivo* can only be predicted. Additional studies *in vitro* will help develop more definitive ways to evaluate this new hypothesis.

In support of histological and cell culture observations, genetic studies also implicate Aβ as a primary event in the pathogenesis of AD (see Cotman & Pike, 1994 for discussion). For example, studies of particular families afflicted with heritable forms of pre-senile AD suggest that the disease is linked with mutations adjacent to the Aβ region of the Aβ precursor protein. In some families, a double mutation is found at APP_{770} 670/671 (Lys-Met to Asn-Leu) just upstream of Aβ (81,81), and single mutations of APP_{770} 717 (Val to Phe, Ile, or Gly) just beyond the Aβ C-terminus are associated with AD in other families (Chartier-Harlin et al., 1991; Goate et al., 1991; Murrell et al., 1991). Such mutations may alter the production, trafficking, storage, or proteolysis of either APP or Aβ. Disruptions to such pathways, however minor, that ultimately yield a net increase in the level of Aβ would be expected to be associated with an increased risk for the development of AD. Consistent with this hypothesis, recent data have demonstrated that the APP 670/671 mutation significantly elevates the secretion of soluble Aβ *in vitro* (Cai et al., 1993; Citron et al., 1992).

CONCLUSION

In many individuals aging compromises behavioral plasticity, the ability to learn and recall information, and to control meaningful changes in behavior. Molecular and cellular plasticity mechanisms, however, serve to provide resilience, offset minor insults, preserve function, and prevent neuronal loss. It is important to identify and strengthen these mechanisms in order to extend not only life, but also the quality of life.

In this chapter we have illustrated the manner in which select molecular and cellular plasticity mechanisms operate in the mature and aged brain to maintain function as neurons become dysfunctional and degenerate. As some neurons lose connections and eventually die, their healthy neighbors grow new processes and regenerate functional synapses. In animal models, for example, a partial lesion of a particularly vulnerable area of the cortex (entorhinal cortex) stimulates the neighboring neurons to grow and resume cortical-hippocampal connectivity and neurotrophic interactions, a process vitally important to the health of neurons. Entorhinal neurons also degenerate with aging and at a greatly accelerated rate in AD. Animal models provided data suggesting that neurons in the brain of AD patients can also regenerate, a prediction confirmed in studies of AD tissue.

AD is not a disease of sudden failure, but one where regeneration and degeneration coexist in a kind of struggle for cellular survival. Regenerative growth appears to help preserve function in the wake of neuronal degeneration and is an example of functional adaptive plasticity. As the disease progresses, however, some of the mechanisms working to fight dysfunction are drawn into a pathological role, particularly senile plaque formation. Senile plaques, with their central core of β-amyloid, grow and mature as the disease progresses. Attracted by β-amyloid and select neurotrophic factors, neurites begin to grow into these structures where they break down and degenerate. At various sites and disease stages β-amyloid appears to function as a neurotrophic retraction factor, a stimulus to neurite degeneration, a risk factor to other insults (e.g., seizures and ischemia), and over time as a stimulus for the cell to program its own death. In this way and others, β-amyloid plays a complex part as an organizing force driving dysfunctional plasticity, perhaps acting in concert with various other molecules at different times.

Recently, genetic studies have identified another arm of the cascade and another risk factor, apolipoprotein E (Apo E), a cholesterol transport protein (Corder et al., 1993). Apo E in the body comes in three variants (E2, E3, and E4) and different individuals carry different combinations of these variants. Those with Apo E4 have a significantly greater risk of developing AD with aging. Moreover, the brains of those carrying genes homozygous for E4 appear to contain significantly more plaques than those with E3 or E2, suggesting that E4 may help drive plaque formation. Indeed, there is evidence that Apo E4 binds to Aβ and accelerates amyloid fibril formation while Apo E2, for example, enhances Aβ solubilitiy and prevents or delays plaque formation (Strittmatter et al., 1993).

As the brain ages it becomes an increasingly finely balanced system. Although the aged brain has a capacity to compensate for damage and repair itself, the process is limited. Some of the very mechanisms serving in repair can become part of the insidious course of pathology in AD. Sorting out the positive and negative effects of the brain's double-edged chemistry will require significant research on well-characterized human brain tissues in concert with animal models. Indeed, research is yielding major advances in identifying the mechanisms that drive disease. As we illustrated early in this chapter, the identification and management of these events in the early stages of loss will lead to higher function later in the lives of the elderly, thereby increasing both productivity and quality of life (Fig. 6.1, star dashed line). This challenge for basic and clinical studies must be met and indeed is being met.

ACKNOWLEDGMENTS

The author would like to acknowledge Randy Black and Dayna Smyth for their editorial assistance and Harald Asbeck for assitance with figure preparation.

REFERENCES

Alzheimer, A. (1907). A characteristic disease of the cerebral cortex. *Allgemeine Zeitschrift für Psychiatria und Psychisch-Gerichtliche Medizin, 44*, 146–148.

Araujo, D. M., & Cotman, C. W. (1992). β-Amyloid stimulates glial cells *in vitro* to produce growth factors that accumulate in senile plaques in Alzheimer's disease. *Brain Res., 569*, 141–145.

Baird, A. and Bohlen, P. (1991). Fibroblast growth factors. In M. B. Sporn and A. B. Roberts (eds.) Peptide Growth Factors and Their Receptors I. New York: Springer-Verlag, pp. 369–418.

Cai X-D, Golde TE, Younkin SG. (1993). Release of excess amyloid *b* protein from a mutant amyloid *b* protein precusor. *Science, 259*, 514–516.

Cajal, R. S. (1928). *Degeneration and regeneration of the nervous system (translated by R. M. May)*. London: Oxford University Press.

Chartier-Harlin M-C, Crawford F, Houlden H, et al. (1991). Early-onset Alzheimer's disease caused by mutations at codon 717 of the b-amyloid precursor protein gene. *Nature, 353*, 844–846.

Citron M, Oltersdorf T, Haass C, et al. (1992). Mutation of the *b*-amyloid precursor protein in familial Alzheimer's disease increases *b*-protein production. *Nature, 360*, 672–674.

Copani, A., Koh, J., & Cotman, C. W. (1991). β-amyloid increases neuronal susceptibility to injury by glucose deprivation. *NeuroReport, 2*, 763–765.

Cotman, C.W. (1989). Synaptic plasticity vs. pathology in Alzheimer's disease: Implications for transplantation. In: *Neuronal Grafting and Alzheimer's Disease*, (Gage, Privat, and Christen, eds.), Springer-Verlag, New York, 54–62.

Cotman, C.W. (1990). Synaptic plasticity, neurotrophic factors, and transplantation in the aged brain. In: *Handbook of the Biology of Aging, Third Edition* (Schneider, E.L., and Rowe, J.W., eds.) Academic Press, San Diego, 255–274.

Cotman, C. W., & Anderson, A. J. (in press). Retention of Function in the Aged Brain: The Pivotal Role of Aβ. In: *Center for Learning and Memory*.

Cotman, C.W., Gomez-Pinilla, F., & Kahle, J.S. (in press). Neural plasticity and regeneration. In: *Basic Neurochemistry: Molecular, Cellular, and Medical Aspects*.

Dipasquale, B., Marini, A. M., & Youle, R. J. (1991). Apoptosis and DNA degradation induced by 1-methyl-4-phenylpydridinium in neurons. *Biochem. Biophys. Res. Comm., 181*, 1442–1448.

Geddes, J. W., Anderson, K. J., & Cotman, C. W. (1986). Senile plaques as aberrant sprout-stimulating structures. *Exp. Neurol., 94*, 767–776.

Geddes, J. W., Monaghan, D. T., Cotman, C. W., Lott, I. T., Kim, R. C., & Chui, H. C. (1985). Plasticity of hippocampal circuitry in Alzheimer's disease. *Science, 230,* 1179–1181.

Goate A, Chartier-Harlin M-C, Mullan M, et al. (1991). Segregation of a missense mutation in the amyloid precursor protein gene with familial Alzheimer's disease. *Nature, 349,* 704–706.

Gomez-Pinilla, F., Cummings, B. J., & Cotman, C. W. (1990). Induction of basic fibroblast growth factor in Alzheimer's disease pathology. *NeuroReport, 1*(3 & 4), 211–214.

Gomez-Pinilla, F., Lee, J. W., & Cotman, C. W. (1992). Basic FGF in adult rat brain: cellular distribution and response to entorhinal lesion and fimbria-fornix transection. *J. Neurosci., 12*(1), 345–355.

Hoyer, S., Oesterreich, K., & Wagner, O. (1988). Glucose metabolism as the site of the primary abnormality in early-onset dementia of Alzheimer type? *J. Neurol., 235,* 143–148.

Hyman, B. T., Kromer, L. J., & Van Hoesen, G. W. (1987). Reinnervation of the hippocampal perforant pathway zone in Alzheimer's disease. *Ann. Neurol., 21,* 259–267.

Hyman, B. T., Van Hoesen, G. W., & Damasio, A. R. (1990). Memory-related neural systems in Alzheimer's disease. *Neurol., 40,* 1721–1730.

Hyman, B. T., Van Hoesen, G. W., Damasio, A. R., & Barnes, C. L. (1984). Alzheimer's disease: Cell-specific pathology isolates the hippocampal formation. *Science, 225,* 1168–1170.

James, W. (1890). *The Principles of Psychology.* New York: Holt.

Kahle, J.S., Ulas, J., & Cotman, C.W. (1993). Increased sensitivity to adenosine in the rat dentate gyrus molecular layer two weeks after partial entorhinal lesions. *Brain Research, 609,* 201–210.

Koh, J. Y., Yang, L. L., & Cotman, C. W. (1990). β-amyloid protein increases the vulnerability of cultured cortical neurons to excitotoxic damage. *Brain Res., 533,* 315–320.

Loo, D.T., Copani, A., Pike, C.J., Whittemore, E.R., Walencewicz, A.J., & Cotman, C.W. (1993). Apoptosis is induced by β-amyloid in cultured central nervous system neurons. *Proceedings in National Academy of Science, 90,* 7951–7955.

Mattson, M. P., Cheng, B., Davis, D., Bryant, K., Lieberberg, I., & Rydel, R. E. (1992). b-amyloid peptides destabilize calcium homeostasis and render human cortical neurons vulnerable to excitotoxicity. *J. Neurosci., 12*(2), 376–389.

Mattson, M. P., Cheng, B., Davis, D., Bryant, K., Lieberberg, I., & Rydel, R. E. (1993). Evidence for excitoprotective and intra-neuronal calcium-regulating roles for secreted forms of the beta-amyloid precursor protein. *Neuron, 10*(2), 243–254.

McKee, A. C., Kosik, K. S., & Kowall, N. W. (1991). Neuritic pathology and dementia in Alzheimer's disease. *Ann. Neurol., 30*(2), 156–165.

Milward, E. A., Papadopoulos, R., Fuller, S. J., Moir, R. D., Small, D., Beyreuther, K., & Masters, C. L. (1992). The amyloid protein precursor of Alzheimer's disease is a mediator of the effects of nerve growth factor on neurite growth. *Neuron, 9*(1), 129–137.

Monyer, H., & Choi, D. W. (1988). Morphinians attenuate cortical neuronal injury induced by glucose deprivation *in vitro. Brain Res., 446*, 144–148.

Murrell J., Farlow M., Ghetti B., & Benson M. D. (1991). A mutation in the amyloid precursor protein associated with hereditary Alzheimer's disease. *Science,* 254, 97–99.

Orrenius, S., McConkey, D. J., Bellomo, G., & Nicotera, P. (1989). Role of Ca++ in toxic cell killing. *TiPS, 10*, 281–285.

Pike, C. J., Burdick, D., Walencewicz, A., Glabe, C. G., & Cotman, C. W. (1992a). b-Amyloid and neurodegeneration *in vitro*: evidence for a role of peptide aggregation. *J. Neurosci., 13*(4), 1676–1687.

Pike, C. J., Cummings, B. J., & Cotman, C. W. (1992b). b-amyloid induces neuritic dystrophy in vitro: similarities with Alzheimer pathology. *NeuroReport, 3*, 769–772.

Pike, C. J., Walencewicz, A. J., Glabe, C. G., & Cotman, C. W. (1991a). Aggregation-related toxicity of synthetic β-amyloid protein in hippocampal cultures. *Euro. J. Pharm., 207*, 367–368.

Pike, C. J., Walencewicz, A. J., Glabe, C. G., & Cotman, C. W. (1991b). In vitro aging of β-amyloid protein causes peptide aggregation and neurotoxicity. *Brain Res., 563*, 311–314.

Quon, D., Catalano, R., & Cordell, B. (1990). Fibroblast growth factor induces beta-amyloid precursor mRNA in glial but not neuronal cultured cells. *Biochem. Biophys. Res., 167*, 96–102.

Schubert, D., Jin, L. W., Saitoh, T., & Cole, G. (1989). The regulation of amyloid beta protein precursor secretion and its modulatory role in cell adhesion. *Neuron, 3*, 689–694.

Stopa, E. G., Gonzalez, A., Chorsky, R., Corona, R. J., Alvarez, J., Bird, E. D., & Baird, A. (1990). Basic fibroblast growth factor in Alzheimer's disease. *Biochem. Biophys. Res. Comm., 171*(2), 690–696.

Strittmatter WJ, Saunders AM, Schmechel D, et al. (1993). Apolipoprotein E: high-avidity binding to b-amyloid and increased frequency of type 4 allele in late onset familial Alzheimer disease. *Proc. Natl. Acad. Sci. USA, 90,* 1977–81.

Terry, R. D., Maslieh, E., Salmon, D. P., Butters, N., DeTheresa, R., Hill, R., Hansen, L. A., & Katzman, R. (1991). Physical basis of cognitive alterations in Alzheimer's disease: synapse loss is the major correlate of cognitive impairment. *Ann. Neurol., 4,* 572–580.

Whitson, J. S., Glabe, C. G., Shintani, E., Abcar, A., & Cotman, C. W. (1990). β-amyloid protein promotes neuritic branching in hippocampal cultures. *Neurosci Lett, 110*(3), 319–24.

Whitson, J. S., Selkoe, D. J., & Cotman, C. W. (1989). Amyloid beta protein enhances the survival of hippocampal neurons in vitro. *Science, 243*(4897), 1488–90.

Wieloch, T. (1985). Hypoglycemia-induced neuronal damage prevented by an N-methyl-D-aspartate antagonist. *Science, 230,* 681–683.

Wyllie, A. H., Kerr, J. F. R., & Currie, A. R. (1980). Cell death: the significance of apoptosis. *Intl. Rev. Cytol., 68,* 251–306.

Yankner, B. A., Duffy, L. K., & Kirschner, D. A. (1990). Neurotrophic and neurotoxic effects of amyloid β-protein: reversal by tachykinin neuropeptides. *Science, 250,* 279–282.

Yoshida, K., & Gage, F. H. (1991). Fibroblast growth factors stimulate nerve growth factor synthesis and secretion by astrocytes. *Brain Res., 538,* 118–126.

Stress as a Pacemaker of Senescent Neuronal Degeneration, and Strategies to Attenuate Its Impact

7

Robert M. Sapolsky

It is true but bordering on the platitudinous to state that the quality of our present reflects the influences of and interactions among all that came in our past. Yet, we must treat that statement as more than a platitude if we are to understand the aging process, especially the considerable individual variation that emerges in the quality of aging. Aging represents the final manifestation of the interactions of biological and environmental influences, influences which can be extraordinarily persistent, echoing across our years.

My own work, examining the causes of neuron death in the hippocampal region of the brain, represents an example of this. Strikingly, such neuron death can be brought about by exposure to stress, and the extent of cumulative exposure to stress over the lifetime can serve as a pacemaker of the rate of hippocampal neuron loss during senescence. Critically, there is tremendous individual variability in vulnerability to this phenomenon, variability reflecting individual differences in experience stretching back to the first days of life. Thus, while much of the literature concerning stress-induced neuro-degeneration is a grim one, there is contained within it at least some hints of hope and potential intervention.

STRESS, GLUCOCORTICOID PHYSIOLOGY AND PATHOPHYSIOLOGY

A stressor can be defined as an environmental perturbation which throws an organism out of homeostatic balance, and the stress-response as the set of endocrine, neural, metabolic (and so on) adaptations which help restore homeostasis. These definitions would suffice for the many species on earth whose stressors are exclusively physical—hunger, an injury, evading a predator, and so on. But when considering more cognitively complex creatures, above all humans, the definition of a stressor must be expanded to include the anticipation of being thrown out of physical homeostasis (Levine et al., 1989). When such anticipation proves valid, the capacity to mobilize the stress-response by psychological means in advance of a physical stressor is highly adaptive. When such anticipation is invalid and occurs often, we might typically describe it as "paranoia," "anxiety," "neurosis," or "hostility."

A cornerstone of stress physiology is that widely different stressors provoke a remarkably similar and convergent stress-response. One of the most consistent and important features of the response to a vast array of physical and psychological stressors is the secretion of glucocorticoids (GCs) by the adrenal gland. These hormones are central to the stress-response, and to the neurodegeneration to be described in this chapter.

Glucocorticoids are secreted as the final step in an endocrine cascade beginning in the brain. Perception or anticipation of a stressor triggers the release of an assemblage of hypothalamic hormones, the most important among these being corticotropin releasing factor (CRF). Along with the other minor "secretagogs," CRF stimulates pituitary release of ACTH which, in turn, stimulates adrenal secretion of GCs. These steroid hormones then exert a broad array of effects throughout the body which, from a teleological standpoint, are essential to successful adaptation to stress (Munck et al., 1984). Along with sympathetic catecholamines, glucagon and growth hormone, GCs halt the storage of energy, mobilize stored energy, and promote hepatic gluconeogenesis, all as a means to supply energy to muscles which are presumably central to surviving a physical stressor. Closely allied to this effect, GCs work in consort with catecholamines to increase cardiovascular tone, enhancing the delivery of nutrients to exercising muscle. The steroids also inhibit a number of long-term anabolic processes which are superfluous, or even deleterious, in the face of an immediate physical emergency. Thus, GCs contribute to the inhibition, during stress, of digestion, growth, inflammation and reproductive physiology. The steroids are also well-known for their suppression of aspects of immunity. The net result is that GCs help mobilize the stress-response, sharpen it, and prevent aspects of it from overshooting (Munck et al., 1984; Sapolsky 1991). The critical importance of these GC actions is demonstrated by the fact that an absence of these steroids—as seen in an adrenalectomized rat or a human with adrenocortical insufficience—is readily fatal in the face of a severe physical stressor.

Yet these same GC actions, if prolonged, can be highly deleterious, and the pathogenic consequences of GC excess are central to the emergence of numerous stress-related diseases. Essentially, the bulk of GC actions are catabolic, yet must be tolerated in the context of coping with an immediate and transient physical stressor; if such stressors are sufficiently prolonged or repeated, the catabolic effects of the GCs themselves become damaging. Among the deleterious consequences are increased risks of adult-onset diabetes, hypertension, peptic ulceration, osteoporosis, numerous reproductive dysfunctions, and immune suppression (Krieger, 1982; Sapolsky, 1991).

Thus, GCs are essential for successful coping with an acute physical stressor, yet the same class of hormone can cause a wide array of pathologies if secreted in excess. It is the latter potential to be pathogenic which must be appreciated in considering how GCs damage neurons of the aging hippocampus.

STRESS- AND GLUCOCORTICOID-INDUCED DAMAGE TO HIPPOCAMPAL NEURONS

The first experimental evidence of GC-induced neurotoxicity came with the report, in the late 1960's, that pharmacological concentrations of GCs damaged the brain (Aus der Muhlen & Ockenfels, 1969). This report made relatively little impact; this probably reflected its publication in German, and the use of the guinea pig in those studies (a rarely used species in gerontological, endocrine or neurobiological research). As an intriguing aspect of that study, damage was found to occur preferentially in the hippocampus. This anatomical pattern was explained by the publication around that time of the first study mapping steroid receptors in the brain; it demonstrated that the hippocampus is among the principal neural target tissues for GC action, as assessed by its density of corticosteroid receptors (McEwen et al., 1968). Indeed, massive levels of receptors for GCs were found to exist in the hippocampus. Thus, pharmacological concentrations of GCs could damage the hippocampus. Over the last 15 years, a series of studies have shown that GCs play a physiological role in the loss of hippocampal neurons with age.

In one style of study, sustained exposure of the rat to elevated GC concentrations—not artificially high levels but the normal levels incurred during stress—would accelerate hippocampal aging. In the first demonstration of this (Sapolsky et al., 1985), we found that three months of exposure to corticosterone, the predominant GC of rats, caused a pattern of hippocampal degeneration remarkably similar to that seen during aging.

Subsequent studies suggest that the GC-induced neuronal degeneration occurs far earlier than the three-month point utilized in that study. Following 3 weeks of administration of similar high concentrations of corticosterone, there is loss of small interneurons within the hippocampus (McEwen, personal communication), as well as other decrements.

A second body of studies demonstrate that *diminishing* GC exposure can *decelerate* the loss of neurons in the aging hippocampus. In the first demonstration of this, 12-month old rats were adrenalectomized and maintained on extremely low levels of corticosterone (producing circulating corticosterone concentrations below detection by radioimmunoassay). When rats were assessed in old age (at approximately 2 years of age), this manipulation was shown to have prevented the loss of neuron density, the glial hypertrophy, and some of the memory deficits typical of aged rats (Landfield et al., 1981).

Subsequent to that, we investigated whether a behavioral manipulation that caused a long-term diminution in GC secretion could also delay features of hippocampal aging (Meaney et al., 1988, 1991). We studied neonatal handling, a developmental phenomenon in which daily handling of rats for the first few weeks of life produces adults with low basal glucocorticoid concentrations. The particular features of neonatal handling will be discussed towards the end of this chapter. At this point, the salient feature of these studies was that handled animals had decelerated hippocampal aging. This included more hippocampal neurons, more hippocampal corticosteroid receptors, and better hippocampal-dependent cognitive skills than did non-handled controls.

Individually, none of these studies was perfect. For example, adrenalectomy obviously eliminates hormones other than just GCs, making it impossible to conclude that it was the consequent absence of GCs which was neuroprotective in the 1981 study by Landfield et al. Nevertheless, these studies suggest collectively that the extent of GC exposure over the lifetime in the rat can act as an important determinant of the extent of neuron loss in the aging hippocampus.

Implicit in this is the idea that sustained stress should damage the hippocampus as well. This has been shown explicitly in a pair of studies. In one, 18-month old rats were exposed to a repeated footshock paradigm that also induces considerable amounts of anxiety. When examined at two years of age, they had sustained an approximate 25% loss of pyramidal neurons, relative to age-matched non-stressed controls (Kerr et al., 1991). In another study, immobilization or immersion into water of rats for 15 minutes/day for a month led to a significant loss of CA3 and CA4 pyramidal neurons (Mizoguchi et al., 1992). (In an unexpected twist that has not yet been fully explored, such stress-induced neuron loss was demonstratable only in castrated animals.)

All of these studies were carried out with rodents. Three other recent studies, though, suggest that stress and GCs have the potential to damage the primate hippocampus as well. The first involved a wild population of vervet monkeys living in Kenya that had become agricultural pests and, as a result, had been trapped and housed in a primate center in Nairobi (Uno et al., 1990). Dominance hierarchies emerged among the animals and, as is often the case with captive primates, subordinate animals suffered from the stressor of not being able to evade dominant individuals in the small cages. As such, a large number of individuals died of a syndrome suggesting sustained social stress. Upon autopsy, they were found to have multiple gastric ulcers, hyperplastic adrenal cortices, splenic lymphoid depletion, colitis and multiple bite wounds (see Guzman-Flores et al., 1987, for the specific linking of these pathologies to social subordinance among captive vervet monkeys). Upon neuropathological examination, they were found to have a pattern of damage remarkably similar to that seen in rats exposed to sustained stress or GCs. Most damage occured within the CA3 region of the hippocampus. In contrast, control monkeys who were euthanized and matched for post-mortem time showed no such neuropathological markers.

A similar report has emerged concerning tree shrews, in which captive subordinates also often die from syndromes of social stress, and with a pathology similar to that described above for vervet monkeys. Among these primates, as little as 2 weeks of such social stress produced selective hippocampal damage (Uno et al., 1991).

A follow-up study suggested that the GC hypersecretion was the mechanism underlying the neurodegeneration in these instances of primate social stress (Sapolsky et al., 1990). Vervet monkeys were stereotaxically implanted with GC-secreting pellets in one hippocampus and, as a control for the steroidal nature of GCs, cholesterol-secreting pellets in the contralateral hippocampus. Upon post-mortem examination one year later, there were a number of markers of hippocampal degeneration in the GC-treated side: cell layer irregularity, dendritic atrophy, soma shrinkage and condensation, and nuclear pyknosis. Once again, damage was restricted to the CA3 region.

These studies suggest that in both the rodent and the primate, GC excess and stress itself can damage the hippocampus and worsen the functional consequences of hippocampal aging. Interestingly, a complete elimination of GCs (via adrenalectomy) will also damage the hippocampus, preferentially targetting neurons of the dentate gyrus (cf. Sloviter et al., 1989). The maintenance of GC concentrations within the normal physiologic range is accomplished through some immensely complex regulatory circuits (cf. Dallman et al., 1987). The capacity for pathologic over- and undersecretion of GCs to both damage the hippocampus is a testament to the importance of this complex regulation.

Among the functional consequences of the hippocampal neurotoxicity induced by GCs or stress is one with an important implication for aging. While the hippocampus is well-known for its role in learning and memory, it also has a role in neuroendocrine regulation. Specifically, the hippocampus is capable of inhibiting secretion of hormones of the adrenocortical axis. As with most endocrine axes, the adrenocortical system is under negative feedback control, such that an elevation of circulating GC concentrations will inhibit subsequent secretion of hypothalamic secretagogs, ACTH and GCs themselves (Keller-Wood & Dallman, 1984). Within the brain, the hippocampus is one of the more important structures which mediate GC negative feedback signals. It appears to do so by way of a projection via the bed nucleus of the stria terminalis and, from there, on to hypothalamic neurons containing the relevant secretagogs.

As the most explicit manifestation of the hippocampus serving this role, damage to that structure will blunt negative feedback regulation of the adrenocortical axis, causing hypersecretion of the various hormones of the system. (This has been demonstrated in the primate as well, Sapolsky et al., 1991.) The details of GC negative feedback regulation, and the role of the hippocampus in this, are extremely complex and beyond the scope of this chapter (see Jacobson & Sapolsky, 1990, for a lengthy review). The main point, however, is that if the hippocampus is progressively damaged with age, this should produce a tendency towards hypersecretion of the hormones of the adrenocortical axis. This is indeed the case.

When combined with the GC neurotoxicity already discussed, this neuroendocrine role of the hippocampus results in a rather insidious and potentially self-reinforcing pattern. Specifically:

1. Hypersecretion of GCs, in some circumstances, can damage the hippocampus. This is likely to have some role in the loss of neurons typical of the aging hippocampus.
2. Hippocampal damage, under some circumstances, results in a tendency towards GC hypersecretion. This is likely to have some role in the excessive secretion of GCs with age.

These two regulatory facets interact in a feed-forward manner, one which we termed the "glucocorticoid cascade" of hippocampal aging (Sapolsky et al., 1986). The original model also incorporated the fact that excessive GC exposure would down-regulate the numbers of hippocampal corticosteroid receptors. This was thought to have two consequences. First, it was posited to explain the decrease in hippocampal corticosteroid receptor number reported by most investigators (reviewed in McEwen, 1992). Second, this compensatory receptor loss was posited to protect hippocampal neurons for awhile from the GC neurotoxicity, explaining the fact that neuron loss does not emerge progressively with age in the hippocampus (reviewed in Coleman and Flood, 1987).

Since the time of that study, research by a number of investigators has confirmed the general features of it (points "A" and "B" immediately above) while forcing modifications of many of the fine points (reviewed in McEwen, 1992, and in Sapolsky, 1992, chapter 6). It has been shown that there are in fact two classes of hippocampal corticosteroid receptors, which differ dramatically in affinity, function, and vulnerability to down-regulation (Reul & de Kloet, 1985; McEwen et al., 1986) and which are lost to differing extents during aging. It has become clear that stress-induced down-regulation of corticosteroid receptors is a rarer event than thought at the time and to the extent that it does occur, it happens less readily in the aged hippocampus than in the young hippocampus (Eldridge et al., 1989). Thus, the aged hippocampus is less likely to have that as a protective defense in the face of sustained neurotoxic exposure to GCs. In support of that conclusion, the older a rat is, the more likely sustained stress is to cause hippocampal neuron loss (Kerr et al., 1991).

When this model was originally proposed, it was meant to describe an obligatory feature of aging. The most interesting modification forced upon this model since then is that this degenerative cascade is far from obligatory or universal to all aging rats. The instances in which this degeneration can be prevented represents the final and most optimistic part of this chapter.

GLUCOCORTICOID-INDUCED ENDANGERMENT OF HIPPOCAMPAL NEURONS

In seeking to understand how GCs might kill hippocampal neurons, we considered the possibility that the steroids were not, in fact, directly toxic. Instead, the hormones might be merely endangering, disrupting some aspect of hippocampal neuronal function or metabolism. In considering this scenario, we have used the metaphor of GCs placing hippocampal neurons close to the edge of a cliff. Should nothing else deleterious happen to the neuron at that point, the period of GC exposure would pass without dire consequences. However, should the neuron now be challenged with a co-incident insult, even an insult that normally does nothing more damaging to a neuron than, in effect, shoving it forward a few steps, it will now go over the edge of the cliff.

Translated into testable terms, this idea generated the prediction that GCs should compromise the ability of hippocampal neurons to survive various neurological insults, increasing the resultant extent of neuron death. This has now been shown in a variety of models of neurological disease, including epileptic seizures, severe hypoglycemia and hypoxia-ischemia as occurs during cardiac arrest.

Thus, neurological diseases that damage the hippocampus become even more damaging in an individual who has been under a lot of stress at the time of the disaster. GCs endanger hippocampal neurons in a broad manner, impairing their ability to survive a variety of insults. The ability of adrenalectomy to reduce hippocampal damage following these insults suggests that the GC stress-response induced by these insults (which is typically massive; Feibel et al., 1977; Stein & Sapolsky, 1988) is sufficient to exacerbate damage. Therefore, what is viewed as "normal" amounts of hippocampal damage after a neurological insult may well be normal amounts augmented by the co-incident endangering effects of high GC concentrations.

Some features of this GC endangerment are now understood. Potentially, the GC endangerment could be secondary to the vast number of effects that these hormones exert throughout the rest of the body. However, this appears to be a direct effect, in that GCs will also enhance excitotoxic, ischemic and hypoglycemic damage to cultured hippocampal neurons and glia (Sapolsky et al., 1988; Tombaugh et al., 1992, 1993).

This direct GC action suggests that it is mediated by interaction with corticosteroid receptors, and indeed this is the case.

Finally, these studies also demonstrate that high concentrations of such GC receptors are neccesary but not sufficient to cause a synergy between GCs and these toxic insults. Instead, those neurons must be particularly sensitive to the insult as well. As evidence, there are plentiful quantities of GC receptors throughout the hippocampus (McEwen et al., 1986). However, the insult/GC synergy is always most pronounced in the hippocampal cell region most sensitive to the insult itself: CA3 for kainic acid, CA1 for hypoxia-ischemia, the dentate gyrus for antimetabolite toxins.

THE CELLULAR MECHANISMS UNDERLYING GLUCOCORTICOID ENDANGERMENT

How then do GCs endanger hippocampal neurons? They appear to exacerbate various steps in a damaging cascade of events let loose during hypoxia-ischemia, seizure and hypoglycemia. During these insults, there is excessive accumulation in the synapse of a class of neurotransmitters called excitatory amino acids (EAAs). The best known of these is glutamate. EAAs trigger the accumulation of calcium in the cytoplasm of neurons and when such levels become pathologically high, calcium can trigger a variety of damaging events in neurons, including the formation of oxygen radicals and the destruction of cell membranes and structural proteins (cf. Choi, 1990).

GCs exacerbate numerous steps in this process (discussed in detail in Sapolsky, 1994):

a) An insult such as a seizure causes EAA accumulation in the synapse and this accumulation is worsened by GCs (Stein-Behrens et al., 1992). Moreover, stress itself will cause such EAA accumulation (Moghaddam, 1993). This accumulation could be due to more EAAs being released into the synapse or less being removed. Our work indicates that GCs predominately disrupt the latter step (Virgin et al., 1991; Chou et al., 1994).

b) If GCs exacerbate EAA accumulation, they should do the same to EAA-induced calcium accumulation in neurons during neurological insults. We have observed this to be the case (Elliot & Sapolsky, 1992). Once again, this could be due to GCs increasing the amount of calcium mobilized into the cytoplasm and/or decreasing the amount removed. The GC effect appears to be more on the removal (Elliot & Sapolsky, 1993).

c) If GCs exacerbate calcium accumulation during insults, calcium-dependent degenerative events should also be worsened. This is observed. For example, GCs exacerbate the degradation of neuronal cytoskeletal (one such calcium-dependent event) following seizures (Elliot et al., 1993).

Why should GCs be able to alter so many features of the EAA/ calcium cascade? Potentially, the hormones might be interacting with some element in this cascade directly—for example, directly antagonizing the activity of the glial glutamate uptake pump. However, our evidence suggests that GCs disrupt these various steps in the cascade through indirect, energetic means.

A common theme among all of these neurological insults made more damaging by GCs is that they constitute energy crises for neurons. Hypoxia-ischemia and hypoglycemia, for example, disrupt energy production, while seizure places a pathologically elevated demand for energy on neurons. All of these insults cause a decline in ATP and phosphocreatine concentrations in the neuron, and their toxicities can be buffered by energy supplementation of the neuron (in the case of hypoxia-ischemia and if it involves glucose, only following the insult) (Auer & Siesjo, 1988; Beal 1992; Sapolsky 1992b).

This common theme of energy disruption among these insults suggested to us that the metaphorical "cliff" which GCs place neurons on the edge of is an energetic one; by somehow disrupting neuronal energetics, GCs made the cells less likely to survive the insults. Were this the case, the GC endangerment of the hippocampus should be reversible with energy supplementation, and this has been shown both *in vivo* (Sapolsky, 1986b) and *in vitro* (Sapolsky et al., 1988), using glucose, mannose and ketones.

What is the mechanism by which GCs endanger the neurons energetically? The hormones have long been known to decrease glucose transport in various peripheral tissues, both via inhibition of transcription of the gene for the glucose transporter, and by causing translocation of pre-existing glucose transporter molecules from off of the cell surface (cf. Horner et al., 1987; Garvey et al.,1989). This catabolic GC action is viewed as part of the general strategy of energy mobilization during an emergency. By inhibiting glucose entry into fat cells, fibroblasts, and so on, energy is diverted indirectly to exercising muscle (Munck, 1971). The hormones turn out to have similar effects in the brain. They decrease glucose utilization in the hippocampus (Kadekaro et al., 1989), and accomplish this by impairing glucose entry into both cultured hippocampal neurons and glia (Horner et al., 1990; Virgin et al., 1991). As would be hoped for—should this effect help explain the GC endangerment—the inhibition of glucose transport in hippocampal neurons by GCs shows the same receptor- and steroid-specificity as does the GC endangerment of these neurons. The inhibition of glucose transport is far less dramatic than in peripheral tissue, in which glucose transport can be inhibited by as much as 70% by GCs (Munck, 1971). Instead, the inhibition is on the order of 20–30%. This is insufficient to kill neurons outright, or to depress their ATP concentrations under non-stressed conditions (unpublished). However, it impairs the capacity of these neurons to cope with an energetic crisis. As evidence, the decline in ATP concentrations in hippocampal glia during hypoxia is accelerated (Tombaugh & Sapolsky 1992), as is the decline in metabolism of neuronal/glial cultures following hypoxia (Lawrence & Sapolsky, 1994).

This mild energy problem for the hippocampus is likely to explain why the various steps of the EAA/calcium cascade are worsened by GCs. The magnitude of the cascade is profoundly sensitive to energy availability. A depletion of energy stores will: a) depolarize neurons, enhancing EAA release, b) compromise the ability of the energetically-costly reuptake pumps to remove EAAs from the synapse, c) enhance the influx of calcium into the post-synaptic cytosolic pool, and d) compromise the efficacy of the energetically-costly sequestering and efflux mechanisms that would normally remove calcium from the neuron. As evidence that it is the energy problem induced by GCs which underlies the GC endangerment, energy supplementation will reverse the GC actions upon EAA accumulation, upon EAA removal from the extracellular space, upon calcium mobilization and upon calcium-dependent degenerative events (Stein-Behrens et al., 1992; Virgin et al., 1991; Elliott & Sapolsky, 1992; Elliott et al., 1993).

Thus, our current model of how GCs endanger the hippocampus is via an energetic route. By curtailing the entry of glucose into neurons and glia, GCs cause these cells to be less capable of the costly task of containing the damaging floods of EAAs and calcium during neurological disease. It should be noted that this model does not imply that this is the sole mechanism of energetic disruption by GCs, or that there are no non-energetic mechanisms as well.

GLUCOCORTICOID ENDANGERMENT OF HIPPOCAMPAL NEURONS: DOES IT APPLY TO GLUCOCORTICOID KILLING OF NEURONS DURING AGING?

As little as 12 hours of GC exposure bracketing the time of a seizure is sufficient to enhance hippocampal damage (Sapolsky, 1986). In contrast, it appears to take weeks of high GC exposure to begin to kill hippocampal interneurons, and months to kill pyramidal cells. Does the model just presented regarding how GCs *endanger* hippocampal neurons during the crisis period immediately surrounding a massive neurological disaster tell us anything about how GCs, in this much longer time-span, gradually *kill* hippocampal neurons during aging?

Part of the answer to this question involves how often the aging hippocampus undergoes minor versions of some of the neurological insults discussed. If, for example, a rat is fed a few hours later than usual for some reason, will the resultant mild hypoglycemia alter EAA/calcium trafficking in a way that is similar to, although milder than, what occurs after severe hypoglycemia? Is a transient bout of cerebral vasospasm, on a cellular level, ischemia writ small? If the answer is yes in these sorts of scenarios, then an excess of GCs may exacerbate these minor crises as well, causing three neurons to die after a mild hypoglycemic episode, rather than the usual two.

If true, GCs may never actually kill neurons directly, even during the gradual course of aging, but may always be endangering instead, impairing the capacity of neurons to survive mild, everyday insults. It would be extremely difficult to determine just how often mild neurological challenges occur during the course of normative aging, let alone whether such incidences are influenced by the GC milieu at that time. This type of problem permeates much of gerontological research. In effect, how often does an age-related decline in function reflect true intrinsic aging (i.e., a smooth decline of function over time), and how often the result of repeated hits by mild (even experimentally undetectable) external insults (i.e., a decline in tiny decremental steps)? For most physiological systems, this question remains unanswerable at present.

It may not be neccesary for the aging hippocampus to undergo mild neurological insults with some regularity for the mechanisms of GC endangerment to be relevant to GC killing. In reviewing the interactions between GCs and the trafficking of EAAs and calcium, the repeated theme was one of GCs augmenting the waves of EAAs and calcium associated with a neurological insult. Do GCs alter EAA or calcium profiles in the absence of an overt insult? In many of the steps in these cascades studied, the answer is no. The effects of GCs, already discussed, upon aspartate accumulation in the synapse, upon calcium efflux, and upon calcium-dependent degenerative events were demonstrable only during neurological crisis such as seizure (Stein-Behrens et al., 1992; Elliott & Sapolsky, 1993; Elliott et al., 1993). In other words, exposure to high GC concentrations exaggerated the response of those measures to seizure, but did not change these variables in the absence of a co-incident neurological insult.

However, some facets of this system might be altered by GCs under even basal conditions, in the absence of an insult. In our microdialysis studies, GC treatment caused a significant elevation of extracellular glutamate concentrations, even *prior* to the induction of a seizure in the rat with kainic acid (Stein-Behrens et al., 1992). Moreover, in our *in vitro* studies, GC exposure enhanced free cytosolic calcium concentrations in neurons, even in the *absence* of an excitotoxic insult (Elliott & Sapolsky, 1993). Finally, in their studies of hippocampal slices, Kerr and colleagues (1989) observed that GCs enhance calcium-dependent afterhyperpolarization, in the absence of any sort of insult. Thus, GCs and stress might activate aspects of the damaging EAA/calcium cascade, rather than merely exacerbate this cascade when it is already activated by a co-incident neurological insult.

There are two caveats in interpreting those findings. First of all, the microdialysis studies involved rats which had undergone a co-incident neurological insult, namely the traumatic insertion of a dialysis probe into the hippocampus. Furthermore, any *in vitro* study can be extrapolated to the *in vivo* realm only with caution. Nevertheless, two more physiological studies already cited support the model that stress and GCs themselves might activate the EAA/calcium cascade of neuron death. These involve awake rats with chronically implanted probes and show that stress enhances extracellular EAA concentrations in the hippocampus (Moghaddam, 1993), and triggers NMDA-mediated increases in hippocampal metabolism (Krugers et al., 1992).

Thus, GCs may not just endanger the aging hippocampus (i.e., exacerbate micro-neurological insults), but may kill outright. Furthermore, this potential may become more pronounced with time: as noted earlier, McEwen and colleagues (personal communication) have observed that 3 weeks of exposure to physiological but elevated GC concentrations will kill interneurons in the hippocampus, suggesting a particular vulnerability on the part of interneurons. These GABA-ergic interneurons typically exert an inhibitory role upon the principal excitatory pyramidal cells, and selective damage to such interneurons are felt by many to predispose neighboring pyramidal cells to epileptogenic hyperexcitation (Balcar et al., 1978; Bakay & Harris, 1981; Houser et al., 1986; Ribak et al., 1979; Romign et al., 1988). Therefore, once interneuronal damage occurs, GCs and stress may be capable of activating EAA/calcium cascades to an even greater extent than has been observed in the various studies of short-term GC exposure. We are now testing this possibility.

STRATEGIES TO DELAY GLUCOCORTICOID-INDUCED HIPPOCAMPAL DAMAGE DURING AGING

When first proposing the "glucocorticoid cascade" model of hippocampal aging (Sapolsky et al., 1986), we suggested that the pathologies and dysfunctions contained within it were likely to be inevitable and normal aspects of rat aging. This was because of the feedforward nature of the loop outlined, in which hippocampal damage could produce GC hypersecretion and GC hypersecretion, in turn, could cause hippocampal damage. Seemingly then, dysfunction of any sort within this dysregulatory loop would be likely to bring about all the other facets of dysfunction.

Pleasingly, this model has had to be revised most emphatically since its original formulation in that this dysfunctional cascade is not inevitable. For example, while there is a tendency towards GC hypersecretion with age among various rat strains (e.g., Fischer 344's, Long-Evans, Sprague Dawleys) (reviewed in Sapolsky, 1991), not all the features of the cascade emerge in all strains.

The GC cascade is also not inevitable among all individuals, even in a rat strain that, in general, shows the degenerative pattern during aging. In the best documented example of this, Issa and colleagues (1990) examined the learning capacity of a population of aged male Long Evans rats with the Morris water maze, comparing them to young controls. As would be expected, there was a significant decrease in performance among the aged animals. And as is typical in such studies, there was a subset (34%) who showed no impairment. Remarkably, those same animals were spared all of the features of the degenerative GC cascade—their GC secretory pattern, profile of hippocampal corticosteroid receptors, and number of hippocampal neurons, were all essentially no different from those of young animals.

What explains this individual variability that gives rise to such "successful agers" and can this knowledge be used strategically to delay aging of this system?

The quality of the neonatal environment appears to be one possible stage of life during which the system can be manipulated. The most striking example of this is seen with neonatal handling, a phenomenon first described more than three decades ago (Levine, 1962). In this paradigm, newborn rats are handled (i.e., picked up and transferred to a new cage for 15 minutes) daily for their first three weeks of life. This induces an array of changes in adrenocortical function in adulthood: rats have lower basal GC concentrations, a faster recovery to baseline at the end of stress and, probably underlying both of those traits, enhanced sensitivity to GC negative feedback (reviewed in Meaney et al., 1991b). The probable cause of the enhanced feedback sensitivity is an imprinting phenomenon that occurs in the hippocampus during the neonatal handling period: there is a permanent increase in the concentration of Type II corticosteroid receptors in that structure, probably mediated by handling-induced changes in thyroid hormone concentrations and, subsequent to that, hippocampal serotonin concentrations (see Meaney et al., 1991b). If neonatally handled rats secrete less GCs as adults, they should be less vulnerable to the GC-induced degenerative changes in the aged hippocampus. Indeed, this is the case (Meaney et al., 1988; 1991). Aged-handled rats were spared the traits constituting the "glucocorticoid cascade" seen in aged non-handled controls: elevated basal GC concentrations, an impaired ability to terminate GC secretion at the end of stress, and a loss of hippocampal pyramidal neurons. Thus, a relatively subtle and transient neonatal manipulation can completely prevent the GC cascade.

At the other extreme, sustained separation of an infant male rat from its mother induces a significant increase in GC secretion and, in a similar but opposite vein to that of neonatal handling, causes a decrease in Type II hippocampal receptors in the hippocampus that persists into adulthood (Seymour Levine, personal communication). It seems quite plausible to speculate then that these are animals which will show more exaggerated versions of the degenerative GC cascade in old age. Such studies are in progress.

Interventions need not be in the neonatal period alone. In the famed environmental enrichment paradigm of Rosenzweig and colleagues, infant rats were shown to develop heavier and thicker cerebral cortices, a greater glia/neuron ratio, more complex dendritic branching in the cortex, more dendritic spines, and more protein synthesis (cf. Rosenzweig et al., 1972). Subsequent work by Diamond and colleagues showed that environmental enrichment during adulthood (and indeed even into old age) could produce similar salutory neuroanatomical and cognitive changes (Diamond, 1988). In a recent study (Mohammed & Seckl, personal communication), environmental enrichment of adults was shown to enhance Type II corticosteroid receptor mRNA levels in the hippocampus. While one must obviously know if this results in more functional receptor (and with what consequences), this intriguing finding suggests that environmental manipulation in the adult can also potentially change the likelihood of some of the facets of the GC cascade emerging during aging.

The manipulations just discussed—manipulations which will alter how readily and robustly a GC stress response is initiated and terminated—focus on the neuroendocrine components of this system. What about manipulations of a psychoendocrine nature, altering whether the organism perceives an event to be stressful in the first place?

To begin with, there is a considerable amount of naturally occurring variability among individuals as to how readily external events are perceived as being stressful enough to provoke GC secretion. For example, a number of strains of rats have been characterized which differ in this parameter. Such animals typically do not differ from wildtype strains in basal GC secretion, or in secretion in the face of major physical stressors. Rather, they differ in their responsiveness to ambiguous, psychological stressors, as well as in their likelihood to develop stress-induced hypertension, to be neophobic, and to learn during such stressors (reviewed in Gentsch et al., 1988). There is also considerable variation among individuals within a strain. In studies of populations of wild baboons living in a national reserve in Kenya, lower basal GC levels were observed among baboons with the most sophisticated competitive social skills. These primates exhibited, among other traits, the greatest ability to discriminate between threatening and neutral situations with rivals, and the greatest degree of social control during tense competitive situations. As an independent cluster of traits, they also had the greatest degree of social affiliation (Sapolsky & Ray, 1988; Ray & Sapolsky, 1992). In humans, classic studies of parents undergoing the stressor of watching their children suffering from cancer, showed lower GC concentrations among individuals with particular coping skills (e.g., a structure of religious rationalization for the disease, an ability to displace anxiety onto smaller, rather than more global features of the disease) (Wolff et al., 1964).

Can manipulations be made in individuals to bring about some of the same coping traits and thus, hopefully, reduce GC secretion in the face of stressors? This is, of course, the province of stress management. Both animal and human studies in this realm have shown the considerable physiologic and pathophysiologic consequences of manipulating perceptions of control, of predictability, of outlets for frustration, and of social support (Weiss, 1972; Rodin 1986; House et al., 1988; Levine et al., 1989; Seligman, 1991). It is clear to me as a physiologist, that it is easier to effectively and safely manipulate the adrenocortical axis through psychological rather than through physiological means.

In conclusion, while an experimental literature suggests a link between exposure to stress and certain features of hippocampal degeneration (as well as with numerous other pathologies), this link is by no means inevitable nor intrinsic to the aging process. Moreover, I suspect that "successful aging" is not merely an attribute of those fortunate individuals who just happen to have the correct phenotype (built on factors ranging from optimal heat shock responses when their cells are stressed to optimal attributional styles when their psyches are stressed). Instead, I believe such salutary states of adaptation can be achieved by many individuals, and that we are gaining increasing knowledge as to how to bring about such states.

REFERENCES

Auer R, Siesjo B 1988 Biological differences between ischemia, hypoglycemia, and epilepsy. *Ann Neurol 24*, 699.

Aus der Muhlen K, Ockenfels H 1979 Morphologische Veranderungen im Diencephalon und Telencephalon nach Storngen des regelkreises Adenohypophyse-Nebennierenrinde III. Ergebnisse beim Meerschweinchen nach Verabreichung von Cortison und Hydrocortison. *Z. Zellforsch, 93*: 126.

Beal M 1992 Does impairment of energy metabolism result in excitotoxic neuronal death in neurodegenerative illnesses? *Ann Neurol, 31*, 119.

Ben-Ari Y 1985 Limbic seizure and brain damage produced by kainic acid: Mechanisms and relevance to human temporal lobe epilepsy. *Neuroscience, 14*: 375.

Brodish A, Odio M 1989 Age-dependent effects of chronic stress on ACTh and corticosterone resposnes to an acute novel stress. *Neuroendocrinology, 49*: 496.

Chiueh C, Nespor S, Rapoport S 1980 Cardiovascular, sympathetic and adrenal cortical responsiveness of aged Fischer–344 rats to stress. *Neurobiol Aging, 1*: 157.

Choi D 1990 Cerebral hypoxia: Some new approaches and unanswered questions. *J Neurosci, 10*: 2493.

Chou Y, Lin W, Sapolsky R 1994 Glucocorticoids increase extracellular aspartate overflow in hippocampal cultures during cyanide-induced ischemia. Brain Research, in press.

Coleman P, Flood D 1987 Neuron numbers and dendritic extent in normal aging and Alzheimer's disease. *Neurobiol Aging, 8*: 521.

Dallman M, Akana S, Cascio C, Darlington D, Jacobson L, Levin N 1987 Regulation of ACTH secretion: Variations on a theme of B. *Recent Prog Horm Res, 43*: 113.

Dellwo M, Beauchene R 1990 The effect of exercise, diet restriction, and aging on the pituitary-adrenal axis in the rat. *Exp Gerontol, 25*: 553.

Diamond M 1988 *Enriching Heredity* Macmillan/Free Press, NY.

Eldridge J, Brodish A, Kute T, Landfield P 1989 Apparent age-related resistance of type II hippocampal corticosteroid receptors to down-regulation during chronic escape training. *J Neurosci, 9*: 3237.

Elliott E, Sapolsky R 1992 Corticosterone enhances kainic acid-induced calcium mobilization in cultured hippocampal neurons. *J Neurochem, 59*: 1033.

Elliott E, Sapolsky R 1993 Corticosterone impairs hippocampal neuronal calcium regulation: Possible mediating mechanisms. *Brain Research*, 1994.

Elliott E, Mattson M, Vanderklish P, Lynch G, Chang I, Sapolsky R 1993 Corticosterone exacerbates kainate-induced alterations in hippocampal tau immunoreactivity and spectrin proteolysis in vivo. *J Neurochem*, 1994.

Erisman S, Carnes M, Takahashi L, Lent S 1990 The effects of stress on plasma ACTH and corticosterone in young and aging pregnant rats and their fetuses. *Life Sci, 47*: 1527.

Garvey W, Huecksteadt T, Lima F, Birnbaum M 1989 Expression of a glucose transporter gene cloned from brain in cellular models of insulin resistance: Dexamethasone decreases transporter mRNA in primary cultured adipocytes. *Mol Endocrinol, 3*: 1132.

Gbadebo D, Hamm R, Lyeth B, Jenkins L, Stewart J, Porter J 1991 Corticosterone's mediation of traumatic brain injury. *Soc Neurosci Abstr, 17*: 65.7

Gentsch C, Lichtsteiner M, Feer H 1988 Genetic and environmental influences on behavioral and neurochemical aspects of emotionality in rats. *Experientia, 44*: 482.

Guzman-Flores C, Alcaraz M, Garcia-Castells E, Ergin F, Juarez J 1987 Estudio experimental de la depresion por estrees social. *Bol Estus Med Biol, 35*: 11.

Hall E 1990 Steroids and neuronal destruction or stabilization. *Steroids and Neuronal Activity*. Wiley, Chicester (Ciba Foundation Symposium 153), p 206.

Hicks S 1955 Pathologic effects of antimetabolites. I. Acute lesions in hypothalamus, peripheral ganglia and adrenal medulla caused by 3-acteylpyridine and prevented by nicotinamide. *Am J Pathol, 31*: 189.

Horner H, Munck A, Lienhard G 1987 Dexamethasone causes translocation of glucose transporters from the plasma membrane to an intracellular site in human fibroblasts. *J Biol Chem, 262*: 17696.

Horner H, Packan D, Sapolsky R 1990 Glucocorticoids inhibit glucose transport in cultured hippocampal neurons and glia. *Neuroendocrinology, 52*: 57.

Hortnagl H, Berger M, Hornykiewicz O 1991 Glucocorticoids aggravate the cholinergic deficit induced by ethylcholine aziridinium in rat hippocampus. *Soc Neurosci Abstracts, 17*: 285.1.

House J, Landis K, Umberson D 1988 Social relationships and health. *Science*, 241: 540.

Ida Y, Tanaka M, Tsuda A 1984 Recovery of stress-induced increases in noradrenaline turnover is delayed in specific brain regions of old rats. *Life Sci, 34*: 2357.

Issa A, Rowe W, Gauthier S, Meaney M 1990 Hypothalamic-pituitary-adrenal activity in aged, cognitively unimpaired rats. *J Neurosci, 10*: 3247.

Jacobson L, Sapolsky R 1991 The role of the hippocampus in feedback regulation of the hypothalamic-pituitary-adrenocortical axis. *Endocr Rev, 12*: 118.

Johnson M, Stone D, Bush L, Hanson G, Gibb J 1989 Glucocorticoids and 3,4-methylenedioxymethamphetamine (MDMA)-induced neurotoxicity. *Eur J Pharmacol, 161*: 181.

Kadekaro M, Masanori I, Gross Pl 1988 Local cerebral glucose utilization is increased in acutely adrenalectomized rats. *Neuroendocrinology, 47*: 329.

Keller-Wood M, Dallman M 1984 Corticosteroid inhibition of ACTH secretion. *Endocr Rev, 5*: 1.

Kerr D, Campbell L, Hao S, Landfield P 1989 Corticosteroid modulation of hippocampal potentials: Increased effect with aging. *Science, 245*: 1505.

Kerr D, Campbell L, Applegate M, Brodish A, Landfield P 1991 Chronic stress-induced acceleration of electrophysiologic and morphometric biomarkers of hippocampal aging. *J Neurosci, 11*: 1316.

Koide T, Wieloch T, Siesjo B 1986 Chronic dexamethasone pretreatment aggravates ischemic neuronal necrosis. *J Cereb Blood Flow Metab, 6*: 395.

Krugers H, Jaarsma D, Korf J, 1992 Rat hippocampal lactate efflux during electroconvulsive shock or stress is differentially dependent on entorhinal cortex and adrenal integrity. *J Neurochem, 58*: 826.

Landfield P, Rose G, Sandles L, Wohlstadter T, Lynch G 1977 Patterns of astroglial hypertrophy and neuronal degeneration in the hippocampus of aged, memory-deficient rats. *J Gerontology, 32*: 3.

Landfield P, Baskin R, Pitler T 1981 Brain-aging correlates: Retardation by hormonal-pharmacological treatments. *Science, 214*: 581.

Lawrence M, Sapolsky R 1994 Glucocorticoids accelerate ATP loss following metabolic insults in cultured hippocampal neurons. Brain Research, in press.

Levine S 1962 Plasma-free corticosteroid response to electric shock in rats stimulated in infancy. *Science, 135*: 795.

Levine S, Coe C, Wiener S 1989 The psychoneuroendocrinology of stress—A psychobiological perspective. In: Levine S, Brush R (eds) *Psychoendocrinology*. Academic Press, New York.

McEwen B 1992 Re-exanination of the glucocorticoid hypothesis of stress and aging. *Progress Brain Res, 93*: 365.

McEwen B, Weiss J , Schwartz L 1968 Selective retention of corticosterone by limbic structures in rat brain. *Nature, 220, 911.*

McEwen B, de Kloet E, Rostene W 1986 Adrenal steroid receptors and actions in the nervous system. *Physiol Rev, 66*: 1121.

Meaney M, Aitken D, Sapolsky R 1991 Postnatal handling attenuates neuroendocrine, anatomical and cognitive dysfunctions associated with aging in female rats. *Neurobiol Aging, 12*: 31.

Meaney M, Viau V, Bhatnager S, Betito K, Iny L, O'Donnell D, Mitchell J 1991b Cellular mechanisms underlying the development and expression of individual differences in the hypothalamic-pituitary-adrenal stress response. *J Steroid Biochem Molec Biol, 39*: 265.

Miller G, Davis J 1991 Post-ischemic surge in corticosteroids aggravates ischemic damage to gerbil CAl pyramidal cells. *Soc Neurosci Abstr, 17*: 302.4.

Mizoguchi K, Kunishita T, Chui D, Tabira T 1992 Stress induces neuronal death in the hippocampus of castrated rats. *Neurosci Lett, 138*: 157.

Moghaddam B 1993 Stress preferentially increases extraneuronal levels of excitatory amino acids in the prefrontal cortex: Comparison to hippocampus and basal ganglia. *J Neurochem*, in press.

Morse J, Davis J 1990 Regulation of ischemic hippocampal damage in the gerbil: Adrenalectomy alters the rate of CAl cell disappearance. *Exp Neurol, 110*: 86.

Munck A 1971 Glucocorticoid inhibition of glucose uptake by peripheral tissues. Old and new evidence, molecular mechanisms and physiological significance. *Perspect Biol MEd, 14*: 265.

Munck A, Guyre P, Holbrook N 1984 Physiological actions of glucocorticoids in stress and their relation to pharmacological actions. *Endocrine Rev, 5*: 25.

Odio M, Brodish A 1988 Effects of age on metabolic responses to acute and chronic strss. *Am H Physiol, 254*: E617.

Oxenkrug G, McIntyre I, Stanley M, Gershon S 1984 Dexamethasone suppression test: Experimental model in rats, and effect of age. *Biol Psychiatry, 19*: 413.

Packan D, Sapolsky R 1990 Glucocorticoid endangerment of the hippocampus: Tissue, steroid and receptor specificity. *Neuroendocrinology, 51*: 613.

Ray J, Sapolsky R 1992 Styles of male social behavior and their endocrine correlates among high-ranking baboons. *Am J Primatology, 28*: 231.

Reul J, de Kloet E 1985 Two receptor systems for corticosterone in rat brain: Microdistribution and differential occupation. *Endocrinology, 117*:L 2505.

Riegle G 1973 Chronic stress effects on adrenocortical responsiveness in young and aged rats. *Neuroendocrinology, 11*: 1.

Rodin J 1986 Aging and health: Effects of the sense of control. *Science, 233*: 1271.

Romijn H, Ruijter J, Wolters P 1988 Hypoxia preferentially destroys GABAergic neurons in developing rat neocortex explants in culture. *Exp Neurol, 100*: 332.

Rosenzweig M, Bennett E, Diamond M 1972 Cerebral effects of differential experience in hypophysectomized rats. *J Comp Physiol Psychol 79*: 56–66.

Sabatino F, Masoro E, McMahan C, Kuhn R 1991 Assessment of the role of the glucocorticoid system in aging processes and in the action of food restriction. *J Gerontol, 46*: B 171.

Sapolsky R 1985 A mechanism for glucocorticoid toxicity in the hippocampus: Increased neuronal vulnerability to metabolic insults. *J Neurosci, 5*: 1227.

Sapolsky R 1985b Glucocorticoid toxicity in the hippocampus: temporal aspects of neuronal vulnerability. *Brain Res, 339*: 300.

Sapolsky 1986 Glucocorticoid toxicity in the hippocampus: Reversal by supplementation with brain fuels. *J Neurosci, 6*: 2240.

Sapolsky 1986b Glucocortiocid toxicity in the hippocampus: Temporal aspects of synergy with kainic acid. *Neuroendocrinology, 43*: 386.

Sapolsky R 1991 Do glucocorticoid concentrations rise with age in the rat? Neurobiol Aging, 13: 171.

Sapolsky R 1992 Neuroendocrinology of the stress-response. In: Becker J, Breedlove S, Crews D, eds. *Behavioral Endocrinology.* MIT Press, Cambridge.

Sapolsky R 1992b *Stress, the Aging Brain, and the Mechanisms of Neuron Death.* MIT Press.

Sapolsky R, Krey L, McEwen B 1983 The adrenocorticla stress response in the aged male rat: impairment of recovery from stress. *Exp Gerontol, 18*: 55.

Sapolsky R, Krey L, McEwen B, Rainbow T 1984 Do vasopressin-related peptides induce hippocampal corticosterone receptors? Implications for aging. *J Neurosci, 4*: 1479.

Sapolsky R, Krey L, McEwen B 1985 Prolonged glucocorticoid exposure reduces hippocampal neuron number: Implications for aging. *J Neurosci, 5*: 1121.

Sapolsky R, Pulsinelli W 1985 Glucocorticoids potentiate ischemic injury to neurons: Therapeutic implications. *Science, 229*: 1397.

Sapolsky R, Krey L, McEwen B 1986a The neuroendocrinology of stress and aging: The glucocorticoid cascade hypothesis. *Endocrine Revs, 7*: 284.

Sapolsky R, Krey L, McEwen B 1986b The adrenocortical axis in the aged rat: Impaired sensitivity to both fast and delayed feedback inhibition. *Neurobiol Aging, 7*: 331.

Sapolsky R, Packan D, Vale W 1988 Glucocorticoid toxicity in the hippocampus: In vitro demonstration. *Brain Res, 453*: 367.

Sapolsky R, Ray J 1988 Styles of dominance and their endocrine correlates among wild baboons (Papio anubis). *Am J Primatol, 18*: 1.

Sapolsky R, Uno H, Rebert C, Finch C 1990 Hippocampal damage associated with prolonged glucocorticoid exposure in primates. *J Neurosci, 10*: 2897.

Sapolsky R, Altmann J 1991 Incidences of hypercortisolism and dexamethasone resistance increase with age among wild baboons. *Biol Psychiatry, 30*: 1008.

Sapolsky R, Zola-Morgan S, Squire L 1991 Inhibition of glucocorticoid secretion by the hippocampal formation in the primate. *J Neurosci, 11*: 3695.

Seligman M 1991 Learned Optimism. Alfred Knopf, New York.

Selye H 1975 Confusion and controversy in the stress field. *J Human Stress, 1*: 37.

Sloviter R, Valiquette G, Abrams G, Ronk E, Sollas A, Paul L, Neubort S 1989 Selective loss of hippocampal granule cells in the mature rat brain after adrenalectomy. *Science, 243*: 535.

Stanton P, Moskal J 1991 Diphenylhydantoin protects against hypoxia-induced impairment of hippocampal synaptic transmission. *Br Res, 546*: 351.

Stein B, Sapolsky R 1988 Chemical adrenalectomy reduces hippocampal damage induced by kainic acid. *Brain Res, 473*: 175.

Stein-Behrens B, Elliott E, Miller C, Schilling J, Newcombe R, Sapolsky R 1992 Glucocorticoids exacerbate kainic-acid-induced extracellular accumulation of excitatory amino acids in the rat hippocampus. *J Neurochem, 58*: 1730.

Theoret Y, Caldwell-Kenkel J, Krigman M 1985 The role of neuronal metabolic insult in organometal neurotoxicity. *Toxicologist, 6*: abstract 491.

Tombaugh G, Sapolsky R Corticosterone accelerates hypoxia-induced ATP loss in cultured hippocmapal astrocytes. *Brain Research, 588*: 154.

Tombaugh G, Sapolsky R Endocrine features of glucocorticoid endangerment in hippocampal astrocytes. *Neuroendocrinology*, in press.

Tombaugh G, Yang S, Swanson R, Sapolsky R 1992 Glucocorticoids exacerbate hypoxic and hypoglycemic hippocampal injury in vitro: Biochemical correlates and a role for astrocytes. *J Neurochem, 59*: 137.

Uno H, Tarara R, Else J, Suleman M, Sapolsky R 1989 Hippocampal damage associated with prolonged and fatal stress in primates. *J Neurosci, 9*: 1705.

Uno H, Flugge G, Thieme C, Johren O, Fuchs E L1991 Degeneration of the hippocampal pyramidal neurons in the socially stressed tree shrew. *Soc Neurosci Abstr, 17*: 52.20.

van Eekelen J, Rots N, Sutanto W, de Kloet E 1991 The effect of aging on stress responsiveness and central corticosteroid receptors in the brown Norway rat. *Neurobiol Aging, 13*: 159.

Vaughan D, Peters A 1974 Neuroglial cells in the cerebral cortex of rats from young adulthood to old age. An electron microscope study. *J Neurocytol, 3*: 405.

Virgin C, Ha T, Packan D, Tombaugh G, Yang S, Horner H, Sapolsky R 1991 Glucocorticoids inhibit glucose transport and glutamate uptake in hippocampal astrocytes: Implications for glucocorticoid neurotoxicity. *J Neurochem, 57*, 1422.

Weiss J 1972 Psychological factors in stress and disease. *Scientific American, 226*: 104.

Wolff C, Friedman S, Hofer M, Mason J 1964 Relationship between psychological defenses and mean urinary 17-hydroxycorticosteroid excretion rates. *Psychosom Med, 26*: 576.

Woolley C, Gould E, McEwen B 1990 Exposure to excess glucocorticoids alters dendritic morphology of adult hippocampal pyramidal neurons. *Brain Res., 531*: 225.

Molecular Approaches to Delay Dysfunction in Later Life

8

Nikki J. Holbrook

INTRODUCTION

Rapid growth in the fields of molecular and cellular biology, as well as advances in biotechnology over the last decade have resulted in a marked increase in our understanding of the bases of various diseases, impacting on both their diagnoses and treatment. Genetic mutations causative for a variety of heritable diseases are being identified at record speed, and developments in recombinant DNA technology have not only led to the production of various gene products for treatment of certain disorders, but more recently have provided the practical means for the treatment or prevention of certain diseases and disabilities through the use of somatic gene therapy.

The last decade has also witnessed considerable progress in our understanding of the processes underlying aging and age-related diseases and dysfunctions. Molecular approaches have been used to identify genes whose expression is altered with age or senescence, as well as to establish the genetic basis for various age-dependent diseases. It is my belief that not only could recombinant DNA technology be employed to produce specific gene products for treatment of age-related disorders, but that somatic gene therapy approaches could soon be utilized for treating or retarding the onset of certain dysfunctions of later life.

This chapter will focus primarily on the potential of gene therapy for combating age-associated diseases and dysfunctions. While it is first necessary to introduce the reader to some basic concepts surrounding this approach, I have tried to keep this general discussion brief. A number of recent more extensive reviews are available on the topic (Anderson, 1992; Crystal, 1992; Miller, 1992; Mulligan, 1993).

GENE THERAPY APPROACHES

Definition and Basic Strategies

Gene therapy refers to the treatment of disease through modification of the cellular genetic program. In most instances research has focused on heritable diseases resulting from mutations that can be corrected by the addition of a functioning gene or its product to the appropriate cells. However, gene transfer can also been used for the purpose of providing cells with a new or enhanced property such as increased immunity against an infectious agent, or an increased ability of host cells to kill tumor cells. This second approach has particular application in the treatment of acquired diseases such as cancer and AIDS.

Current efforts in humans have been restricted to somatic cell therapy in which gene insertion is limited to somatic cells of the body with special care to avoid introduction of exogenous genes into germ cells as these carry the possibility of modifying the gene pool. This is in contrast to "transgenic" approaches utilized in various animal and plant models in which germ-line cells are subjected to genetic manipulation for the purpose of generating offspring carrying a particular gene of interest.

Two basic strategies of gene therapy have been employed. In the first case, termed *ex vivo* gene therapy, cells are removed from an individual, modified *in vitro* to allow insertion of the gene of interest and then subsequently introduced back into an appropriate host. This is most frequently carried out using autologous cells derived from the recipient of the therapy, but can in theory also utilize cells from other donors. In the second strategy, termed *in vivo* gene therapy, cells are modified *in vivo* through the direct transfer of genetic information via vectors. Because of the concern that germ cells of a patient could become modified as a side effect of *in vivo* therapy, all studies with human subjects thus far, have utilized *ex vivo* methods of therapy. However, it is likely that with increased developments in the technology for gene transfer over the next few years, and increased evidence for the safety of such techniques through their use in animal studies, that *in vivo* therapy in humans will increase. Such developments will be necessary for the successful application of gene therapy to many cells and tissues, such as those of the central nervous system, which cannot be removed and propagated *in vitro* as required for *ex vivo* procedures.

Vector Systems for Delivery of Genes

For gene therapy to be successful, the transfer of genetic material to target cells must be highly efficient and expression of the transferred gene be maintained for long periods of time. These two requirements have been roadblocks in early attempts at gene transfer which utilized plasmid vectors and either chemical (e.g., calcium phosphate precipitation) or physical (e.g., electroporation) means for transferring genetic information to recipient cells. However, methods utilizing viral vectors for delivery of genetic material have greatly improved the efficiency of transfer and in certain cases have increased the length of expression. While a variety of different viral vectors are currently available (Mulligan, 1993), retroviral and adenovirus vectors are most frequently used.

Retroviral mediated gene transfer

Retroviruses are RNA viruses which enter cells through specific surface receptors and are then transcribed into DNA. Retroviruses possess two main advantages for gene therapy: 1) a high efficiency of gene transfer into recipient cells, and 2) the ability to integrate the genes they carry into cellular DNA. A major disadvantage of retrovirus vectors is the requirement that treated cells be dividing for the integration and continued expression of transferred genes, thus limiting their use to proliferating cells. Also, there is a risk of insertional mutagenesis resulting from the disruption of the normal expression of a critical gene.

Adenovirus vectors

Adenoviruses are double-stranded DNA viruses that enter cells through an as yet unidentified, but widely expressed receptor. Following infection, the virus sheds its protein coat and enters the host cell nucleus. In contrast to retroviruses, adenoviruses generally do not insert into the genome but rather exist almost exclusively in an extrachromosomal state. Just as for the retroviral vectors, construction of adenovirus vectors involves removal of much of the viral genome to make room for the exogenous gene one wishes to transfer and to render the virus incapable of replicating itself in the recipient cell. Two major advantages of adenovirus vectors are: 1) that they can accommodate much larger pieces of exogenous DNA than can retroviral vectors, and 2) that they do not require that the host cell be capable of dividing for efficient gene transfer and long-term expression. Thus, adenoviruses are likely to find their primary application in *in vivo* gene therapy strategies for organs where the target cells proliferate slowly or not at all. Two disadvantages of adenovirus vectors are: 1) that they contain viral genes that could stimulate immunity against the cells they infect, and 2) impermanency of gene expression since the vector does not stably integrate into the recipient cell genome and is lost from dividing cells.

Other delivery systems

As already mentioned above, a number of gene delivery systems employing physical or chemical means to transfer plasmid vectors expressing foreign genes of interest to receipient cells and tissues have been utilized in animal models. Liposomes, inorganic salts, electroporation, etc. have been used with varying efficiency and success in achieving long-term expression. Surprising success has been obtained by the direct microinjection of DNA into some tissues with both efficient uptake and continued expression of gene constructs observed. More specific cellular targeting has been obtained using complexes containing ligands recognized by cellular receptors. Continued advances in such gene delivery systems are likely to be forthcoming.

Cellular Targets for Gene Therapy

A major consideration in the selection of recipient cells for gene transfer is whether the correction of a given defect requires that the corrective gene be transferred directly into the cells displaying effects of gene deficiency, or whether the gene product can be taken up if made by other cells and secreted into the peripheral circulation.

One of the main targets of gene therapy has been stem cells of the haematopoietic system (reviewed in Miller, 1992). While many groups have achieved transfer and long-term expression of genes in mouse haematopoietic cells, results with larger animals including primates have been less successful. Lymphocytes have provided an alternative vehicle for therapy, and in fact, as discussed by Blaese (1991) offer a number of advantages. Most importantly, if necessary they can be easily removed from the host or donor, genetically modified *in vitro*, expanded and enriched for expression of transferred genes of interest, and then be given back to a patient. Because of the critical role they play in the immune response they are likely to be of increased importance in gene therapy for the treatment of acquired diseases such as cancer and AIDS (Rosenberg, 1992; Anderson, 1992). In fact, human trials currently in progess are evaluating the use of genes encoding tumor necrosis factor (TNF) and/or interleukin–2 to enhance the capability of genetically modified lymphocytes to kill tumor cells.

Other cellular targets currently under investigation include fibroblasts, keratinocytes, hepatocytes, lung epithelial cells, neuronal cells, and both skeletal and vascular smooth muscle cells. It is expected that others will be added to this list as the technology develops.

Human Gene Therapy Trials

Based on promising results obtained with various animal models which suggested both safety and efficacy, the first human gene therapy trials began in 1989. The main purpose of initial trials was to establish that gene transfer could be accomplished safely in humans, and to verify the expression of transferred genes. Over the past 4 years some 20 protocols for gene therapy have received approval for use in humans throughout the world, and more protocols are pending (Anderson, 1992; Miller, 1992). While it will be some time before it is possible to evaluate the results of the various protocols, early results of several of these, most notably the treatment of severe combined immunodeficiency disease (due to a defect in the adenosine deaminase (ADA) gene) with a normal ADA gene, are highly encouraging. We should expect therefore, that the next few years will witness a significant increase in the application of gene therapy to a wide range of diseases.

APPLICATION OF GENE THERAPY APPROACHES TO AGING

While the treatment of human disorders through gene therapy is rapidly becoming a reality, the application of such technology to age-related dysfunctions, with the exception of genetic diseases whose expression is age-dependent, lies in the future. A number of important questions must be addressed.

For example, do we know enough about the aging process to attempt to apply such technology? What genes or physiologic functions should be targeted? Is such an approach practical for the masses (since everyone ages)? And, what are the ethical concerns? Here I will attempt to address such questions in the remainder of this discussion.

Aging: Basic Processes Versus Age-Related Diseases

Human aging is accompanied by a progressive decline in many physiological processes. However, longitudinal studies show striking variations among individuals in the loss or retention of physical and mental functions with aging. These individual differences largely reflect the influences of life-style, diet, disease, and genetic factors on these processes. It appears that such factors, while neither the cause nor direct result of aging, can accelerate or retard the development of diseases and disabilities that accompany chronological age. Because such information is likely to have a bearing on the strategies devised to prevent the occurrence of age-associated dysfunctions, it is imperative that we be able to distinguish between those dysfunctions resulting from basic processes of aging and those which are caused by disease.

Age-related diseases

Age-related diseases with a clear genetic basis represent the most likely candidates for use of gene therapy approaches to delay dysfunction in the aged population. Examples of age-associated diseases for which there is strong evidence of a genetic component are diabetes, cardiovascular disease, certain types of cancer including breast, colorectal, and prostatic, and neurodegenerative disorders including amyotrophic lateral sclerosis (ALS), Huntington's, and Alzheimer's diseases. While in all of these cases a genetic link has been established, for most we are far from understanding the specific genetic defect responsible for their development. For example, although the gene responsible for the development of Huntington's disease has recently been identified, neither its normal cellular function nor the biochemical basis for disease is known (Huntington's Disease Collaborator Research Group, 1993; Goldberg et al., 1993). ALS has been linked to the superoxidedismutase 1 (SOD1) gene which encodes a key protective enyzme which detoxifies oxygen radicals, but it is not yet clear how defects in SOD are manifested in brain degeneration (Rosen et al., 1993). Thus, the genes responsible for causing age-dependent diseases must be isolated and thoroughly characterized. Such characterization is not only necessary before gene therapy approaches could be utilized to combat these diseases, but also will likely offer other strategies for their treatment such as pharmacologic or lifestyle interventions. Alzheimer's disease, the most common cause of dementia in the elderly population, would have to rank among those diseases with the highest priority in this respect. However, this is likely to prove more difficult than might previously have been thought, as it now appears that several genetic loci may be involved in the pathogenesis of various forms of this debilitating disease (St. George-Hyslop et al., 1992; Van Broeckhoven et al., 1992, Wasco, Brook, & Tanzi, 1993; Tanzi et al., 1992). While one of the candidate genes, the amyloid precursor protein, has been studied extensively, its role in the pathogenesis of Alzheimer's disease is still unproven.

Gene therapy approaches might also be utilized for treatment of acquired age-related disorders which lack a clear genetic basis. An example of such a disorder is Parkinson's disease, a neurodegenerative disorder characterized by a loss of midbrain dopaminergic neurons that innervate the striatum. Current treatments for the disease employ pharmacological approaches aimed at augmenting striatal dopamine levels. An alternative strategy currently being explored is the replacement of dopamine neurons in the brain using fetal-cell transplants. An extension of this approach in which muscle cells transfected with the gene encoding tyrosine hydroxylase (which converts tyrosine to L-DOPA) were grafted into the striata has recently been reported to correct the disease in a rat model (Jiao, Gurevich, & Wolff, 1993). If such findings can be supported by others and extended in primate models to demonstrate amelioration of other neurological deficits, they could offer an effective treatment for human Parkinson's disease.

Another very recent development with respect to potential treatment of Parkinson's disease in the future is the cloning of a gene encoding a specific neurotrophic factor, glial cell line-derived neurotrophic factor (GDNF) which promotes the survival and differentiation of midbrain dopaminergic neurons (Lin et al., 1993). The ability to deliver cells expressing this gene product directly to the midbrain could prevent degeneration of the dopaminergic neurons.

Basic processes of aging

The critical processes of aging, are believed to be those occurring in all individuals in the absence of apparent disease. Many theories have been put forth to explain such changes, but in general fall within two major classes: *programmatic* theories maintain that aging is an inherent genetic process, while *stochastic* theories state that aging results from random environmental damage and argue that limitations in the repair of damage is an important cause of aging. Current concepts (reviewed by Martin, Danner and Holbrook, 1993) suggest that aging is multifactorial, resulting from oxidative damage due to generation of free radicals, wear and tear, cellular senescence, programmed cell death, changes in nuclear and mitochondrial DNA, etc., each of which contributes to reducing the performance of cells and tissues. Thus, most likely, aging is both programmed and stochastic, involving both genetic and environmental factors.

Can gene therapy approaches be used to counteract basic aging processes and/or prevent age-related declines in physiologic function? In theory, yes, if particular gene products can be identified whose expression influences the aging process. For example, research in lower organisms such as the nematode, suggest that there are specific genes which influence longevity (Johnson & Lithgow, 1992). If similar genes are also present in humans, they could be manipulated to affect the life span of people. While discussion of the potential use of molecular approaches to increase life span is not the focus of this chapter, similar arguments could be made concerning the control of genes whose products aid in the defense of the organism against stress, and thus impact on the quality of life.

Enhancement of Host Defenses to Stress

My own research has focused on genetic responses to environmental stress (or damage) believing that these might represent key defenses against aging. As mentioned above, current concepts relate declines in physiologic function to the accumulation of damage done to molecules, cells, and tissues by a variety of toxic factors which are either produced endogenously during normal cell growth or derived from the environment. Normal function and even survival is dependent on the ablity of cells to sustain homeostasis via their ability to resist such stress and to repair or replace damaged molecules.

It is not surprising then, that genetic systems have evolved to detect specific forms of damage and to activate the expression of genes whose products increase the resistance of the cell to damage and/or aid in its repair. The types of genes induced are dependent on the nature of the stress. For example, heat stress induces one set of genes, oxidative stress another, and antigenic challenge still another, although there is clearly some overlap in the responses. The continued effectiveness of these genetic responses to environmental damage may be a major factor in the resistance to disease and disabilities of aging. My laboratory, as well as those of others, has provided evidence to suggest that certain of these host defenses do indeed decline with aging. If these defenses are important in combating basic aging processes then their enhancement should improve the ability of individuals to cope with the stresses of everyday life and increase their resistance to disease, thereby decreasing dysfunction in later life. Three such host defense mechanisms I will address below include the immune response, anti-oxidant defenses, and heat shock proteins. In all three cases the goal of gene therapy would be to enhance the functional properties of cells (heighten these defenses) such as is currently being evaluated in gene therapy trials for treatment of acquired diseases.

Enhancement of immune function

One of the most striking and consistent observations with mammalian aging is a decline in immune competency (Ben-Yehuda & Weksler, 1992). This not only results in a greater susceptibility and vulnerability of aged individuals to infections, but also likely accounts, at least in part, for an increased incidence of cancer in aged individuals relative to young adults. Most declines in immune function appear to be related to impaired T-cell function (Song et al., 1993; Murasko & Goonewardene, 1991). While a number of lymphokines show altered expression during aging, the best characterized change involves decreased expression of the T-cell growth factor, interleukin–2 (IL–2), which plays a key role in the regulation of T-cell functions. IL–2 is present in low levels in quiescent T-cells, but increases markedly in response to antigenic stimulation. Impaired proliferation of cultured T-cells from aged individuals following their stimulation with mitogens and antigens is correlated with decreased ability to produce IL–2 (Nagel et al., 1989; Rabinowich et al., 1985). Addition of exogenous IL–2 restores, at least in part, the proliferative capacity as well as a variety of other immune functions in mice (Thoman & Weigle, 1985). Thus, it seems likely that transfer of the IL–2 gene under the control of a constitutive promoter to aged lymphocytes could be used to enhance immune competency in the elderly, and there is already good evidence from attempts to use this strategy to combat cancer to support this view. For example, infusion of recombinant IL2 has been utilized in combination with other adoptive immunotherapy stategies to enhance immune destruction of tumor cells (Rosenberg, 1992a). While such studies have provided encouraging results, systemic administration of high doses of IL–2 was found to be associated with significant toxicity. In addition, the presence of IL–2 in the peripheral circulation was too short-lived to be practical for the enhancement therapy I suggest here. The ability to transfer the IL–2 gene directly to cells of interest avoids the systemic effects while enhancing immune function. Again, while results utilizing such gene transfer in various animal models and in human cancer patients have been encouraging in that tumor regression is achieved, with few exceptions the disease has been shown to recur (Anderson, 1992; Rosenberg, 1992b). This should not be discouraging with respect to enhancing immune function during aging, however, as the goal is quite different than for treatment of cancer where cure requires virtually total elimination of the already existing tumor cells. That is, 99% elimination of tumor cells will not cure the patient. In addition, human trials utilizing this approach have so far been restricted to patients with the most severe, life-threatening forms of cancer. In contrast, even a small increase in immune function could have an enormous impact on the ability of the aged to resist infection and/or prevent the development of cancer.

Enhancement of host defenses to oxidative stress

Oxidative stress, resulting from the exposure of cells and tissues to "reactive oxygen species," is a major cause of both acute and chronic cell injury. Free radicals generated both endogenously and exogenously have been shown to play an important role in the pathogenesis of many disease states and are believed to contribute directly to the aging process (Warner, 1992). Cells contain a number of anti-oxidant defenses, including enzymes belonging to the superoxide dismutase (SOD) family, glutathione peroxidase family, and catalase, all of which function to detoxify or eliminate free radicals. Several studies have suggested that expression of these anti-oxidant enzymes declines with age, although other studies have failed to show age-related differences (reviewed in Warner, 1992). Whether or not the level of expression of these anti-oxidants actually declines with aging or not, it is presumed that they are not present in levels high enough to block the damage due to free radicals.

A number of studies have provided evidence to suggest that enhanced or overexpression of SOD enzymes can protect cells or tissues against damaging effects of free radicals. Mammals have three distinct SODs: a cytosolic CuZn-SOD, a mitochondrial MN-SOD, and an extracellular SOD. Mutations within the CuZn-SOD gene have been associated with familial ALS (Lou Gehrig's disease), suggesting that free radicals play a role in the development of this age-dependent disease (Rosen et al., 1993). A number of studies have suggested that enhancement of these anti-oxidant defenses through gene therapy could play an important role in protecting aged tissues from the debilitating effects of chronic oxidative stress and perhaps retard the loss of physiologic function that occurs with aging. (Church et al., 1993; Orr & Sohal, 1992; Reveilland et al., 1991; Wispe et al., 1992). However, design of such stategies should consider what cells or tissues would be targeted. Since it is impossible to increase expression in all tisssues without using a transgenic approach, the tissues and particular cell types presumed to be most vulnerable to oxidative stress should be targeted.

Enhancement of heat shock proteins

The most extensively studied host response to acute stress is the expression of the heat shock proteins (HSPs). In fact, the so-called "heat shock response" is the most highly conserved stress response known to the living world, occurring in every organism tested from bacteria to man (Lindquist & Craig, 1988). HSPs are rapidly transcribed and translated in cells and tissues exposed to a variety of stresses, including heat, heavy metals, analogues of amino acids, and certain chemotherapeutic agents. HSPs, often referred to as chaperones, are known to aid in the synthesis, folding and intracellular transport of proteins, as well as facilitate the disassembly and disposal of damaged protein. The beneficial effects of HSPs during stress have been implied by their association with a state of thermotolerance in cultured mammalian cells. For example, a number of thermoresistant cell variants have been shown to express elevated levels of one or more HSPs (Lazlo & Li, 1985; Chretian & Landry, 1988). In addition, over-expression of recombinant HSP70 and HSP27 has been shown to confer heat resistance to cells (Lavoie et al., 1993; Li et al., 1991). Conversely, inhibition of HSP expression results in greater thermosensitivity (Riabowal, Mizzen, & Welch, 1988; Johnston & Lucey, 1988). In a single study *in vivo*, expression of HSP70 protein in rabbit retina following a mild heat stress was correlated with protection of this tissue from subsequent light damage (Barbee et al., 1988). Thus, there is considerable evidence that these proteins protect against various damaging factors, and are part of a protective homeostatic response.

While most of our knowledge concerning the homeostatic role of HSPs has come from studies using cultured cells, it is clear that HSPs are also expressed in the intact animal, and elevated levels have been associated with a number of disease states (Morimoto, Tissieres, & Georgopoulos, 1990). We have demonstrated that HSP70 is induced in rodents in response to milder forms of stress such as restraint or immobilization, and this induction is linked to classical hormone stress response (Blake et al., 1991; Udelsman et al., 1993). These findings indicate that HSPs are expressed in response to a wider array of stresses than previously realized and likely play a fundamental homeostatic role influencing the organism's ability to cope with stress. We and others have now provided considerable evidence that there is a decline in stress-induced HSP gene expression with aging (Blake et al., 1991; Liu et al, 1990; Fargnoli et al., 1991; Heydari et al., 1993; Udelsman et al., 1993). We believe that a general decline in the ability to mount this response renders the aged individual more vulnerable to stress further contributing to the aging process.

Could aging individuals benefit from gene therapy or other

interventions aimed at enhancing the expression of HSPS? While there is currently no direct evidence *in vivo* to support this notion, I believe so. In fact, Heydari et al. (1993) have recently provided evidence that the age-related decline in HSP70 expression that occurs in heat-stressed hepatocytes of rats can be prevented by dietary restriction. With respect to the development of gene therapy approaches to enhance this host defense, as in the case for enhancing anti-oxidant defenses, it must be carefully considered what tissues or cell types would be targeted for gene transfer.

Ethical and Practical Considerations

Gene therapy is subject to a number of ethical and practical considerations as previously reviewed by others (Miller, 1992; Anderson, 1992), and these are further complicated with respect to the use of such therapies to combat the disabilities that accompany aging.

Safety

Since gene therapy trials first began in 1989, the greatest concern has been one of safety. Although there appears to be general agreement that somatic cell gene therapy constitutes an ethical therapeutic option for the treatment of serious diseases, one must consider the benefit to risk ratio for the patient. In some cases of severe disease where death is imminent without intervention, the ratio is high and the choice is easy. In other cases where disease progression is slower and, though debilitating, less life-threatening, the choice is less obvious. This is of particular concern with respect to many of the age-related diseases such as dementia and becomes particularly difficult with respect to enhancement therapies where no particular disease association is obvious. However, it is likely that as more information is gained from on-going trials, many of our concems about safety will be alleviated.

Cost

At present gene therapy is very costly and thus is not practical for treatment of people en masse. However, it is likely
that with certain age-related diseases such as Huntington's or
Alzheimer's disease, where only subpopulations of the aged
community are affected, the cost of gene therapy could in fact
be less than the cost of supportive care currently required for
long periods of time. However, cost becomes a more significant issue with respect to enhancement therapy aimed at
achieving better function in aged life. As we age, all of us are
affected. Who then should be given such treatments, and who
should pay for it?

When should therapy for age-related diseases begin?

Justification for use of gene therapy to treat specific age-related diseases is no different than that currently being used
for treatment of other heritable or acquired diseases. However, the issue of when to begin such treatment must be carefully evaluated. That is, do we begin treatment before any
symptoms are apparent, or only after certain criteria for disease manifestations are met? This is likely to be an important
consideration, and the answer will vary depending on the particular disease, impacting on both the cost and effectiveness
of the treatment.

Is interference with basic aging processes ethical?

This is probably the most difficult question to deal with
and likely to stir considerable debate if enhancement therapies aimed at altering basic processes of aging are seriously
considered. The efficacy of enhancement therapies to increase physiologic functions will have to be clearly established. For example, it must be clear that enhancement of one
physiologic function does not result in increased longevity
with greater disability with respect to another physiologic
function.

SUMMARY

Recent advances in molecular and cellular biology have led to the development of novel treatments for disease through the use of gene therapy. Applications of this approach for the treatment or prevention of at least some age-dependent disorders, such as Parkinson's disease, are likely to occur in the near future. During the time in which this manuscript was in preparation, the genes responsible for three different age-dependent diseases were discovered. These include the susceptibility genes for Huntington's disease (Huntington's Disease Collaborative Research Group, 1993), ALS (Rosen et al., 1993), and familial colorectal cancer (Peltomaki et al., 1993). How long might it be before such information could be transformed into effective gene therapeutic approaches? Obviously, no one can answer such a question with certainty. However, we should be encouraged by the fact that it took less than 4 years from the time the mutant gene responsible for cystic fibrosis was identified to the approval of a gene therapy protocol aimed at its treatment. In contrast to treatment of age-dependent diseases, use of gene therapy for the purpose of altering basic processes of aging is not likely to be vigorously pursued in the near future. However, in the long-term, gene therapy could provide a viable means to prevent or delay the onset of certain age-related dysfunctions.

REFERENCES

Anderson, W.F. (1992). Human gene therapy. *Science 256*: 808–813.

Ben-Yehuda, A., & Weksler, M.E. (1992). Host resistance and the immune system. *Clinics in Geriatric Medicine 8*: 701–71 1.

Blaese, R.M. (1991). Progress toward gene therapy. *Clin. Immunol. Immunopathol. 61*: S47–55.

Blake, M.J., Udelsman, R., Feulner, G.J., Norton, D.D., & Holbrook, N.J. (1991). Stress induced HSP70 expression in adrenal cortex: a glucocorticoid-sensitive, age-dependent response. *Proc. Natl. Acad. Sci. USA 88*: 9873–9877.

Chowdhury, J.R., Grossman, M., Gupta, S., Chowdhury, N.R., Baker,

J.R., Jr., & Wilson (1991). Long-term improvement of hypercholesterolemia after ex vivo gene therapy in LDLR-deficient rabbits. *Science 254*: 1802–1805.

Chretian, P., & Landry, J. (1988). Enhanced constitutive expression of the 27-KDa heat shock proteins in heat-resistant variants from chinese hamster ovary cells. *J. Cell. Physiol. 137*: 157–166.

Church, S.L., Grant, J.W., Ridnour, L.A., Oberley, L.W., Swanson, P.E., Meltzer, P.S., & Trent, J.M. (1993). Increased manganese superoxide dismutase expression suppresses the malignant phenotype of human melanoma cells. *Proc. Natl. Acad. Sci. USA 90*: 3113–3117.

Crystal, R.G. (1992). Gene therapy strategies for pulmonary disease. *Amer. J. Med. 92 (suppl 6A)*: 44S–52S.

Fargnoli, J., Kunisada, T., Fornace, A.J., Jr., Schneider, E.L., & Holbrook, N.J. (1990). Decreased expression of HSP70 MRNA and protein after heat shock in cells of aged rats. *Proc. Natl. Acad. Sci. USA 87*: 846–850.

Goldberg, Y.P., Rommens, J.M., Andrew, S.E., Hutchinson, G.B., Lin, B., et al. (1993). Identification of an Alu retrotransposition event in close proximity to a strong candidate gene for Huntington's disease. *Nature 362*: 370–373.

Heydari, A.R., Wu, B., Takahashi, R., Strong, R., & Richardson, A. (1993). Expression of heat shock protein 70 is altered by age and diet at the level of transcription. *Mol. Cell. Biol. 13*: 2909–2918.

Huntington's Disease Collaborative Research Group. (1993). A novel gene containing a trinucleotide repeat that is expanded and unstable on Huntington's disease chromosomes. *Cell 72*: 971–983.

Jiao, S., Gurevich, V., & Wolff, J.A. (1993). Long-term correction of rat model of Parkinson's disease by gene therapy. *Nature 362*: 450–453.

Johnson, T.E. & Lithgow, G.J. (1992). The search for the genetic basis of aging: the identification of gerontogenes in the nematode Caenorhabditis elegans. *J. Amer. Geriat. Soc. 40*: 936–945.

Johnston, R.N., & Lucey, B.L. (1988). Competitive inhibition of HSP70 gene expression causes thermosensitivity. *Science 242*: 1551–1554.

Lavoie, J.N., Gingras-Breton, G., Tanguay, R.M., & Landry, J. (1993). Induction of Chinese hamster HSP27 gene expression in mouse cells confers resistance to heat shock. *J. Biol. Chem. 268*: 3420–3429.

Lazlo, A., & Li, G.C. (1985). Heat-resistant variants of chinese hamster fibroblasts altered in expression of heat shock protein. *Proc. Natl. Acad. Sci. USA 82*: 8029–8033.

Li, G., Ligeng, L., Liu, Y., Mak, J.Y., Chen, L., & Lee, W.M.F. (1991). Thermal response of rat fibroblast stably transfected with the human 70 KDa heat shock protein-encoding gene. *Proc. Natl. Acad. Sci. USA 88*: 1681–1685.

Lin, L.-F. H., Doherty, D.H., Lile, J.D., Bektesh, S., & Collins, F. (1993). GDNF: A glial cell line-derived neurotrophic factor for midbrain dopaminergic neurons. *Science 260*: 1130–1132.

Lindquist, S., & Craig, E.A. (1988). The heat-shock proteins. *Annu. Rev. Genet. 22*: 631–677.

Liu, A.Y.C., Lin, Z., Choi, H.S., Sorhage, F., & Li, B. (1989). Attenuated induction of heat shock gene expression in aging diploid fibroblasts. *J. Biol. Chem. 264*: 12037–12045.

Martin, G.R., Danner, D.B., & Holbrook, N.J. (1993). Aging—causes and defenses. *Annu. Rev. Med. 44*: 419–29.

Miller, A. D. (1992). Human gene therapy comes of age. *Nature 357*: 455–460.

Morimoto, R.I., Tissieres, A., & Georgopoulos, C. (1990). *Stress Proteins in Biology and Medicine*. R.I. Morimoto, A. Tissieres, C. Georgopoulos, eds. Cold Spring Harbor Press, Cold Spring Harbor, NY.

Mulligan, R.C. (1993). The basic science of gene therapy. *Science 260*: 926–932.

Murasko, D.M., & Goonewardene, I.M. (1990). T-cell function in aging: mechanisms of decline. *Annu. Rev. Gerontol. Geriat. 10*: 71–96.

Nagel, J.E., Chopra, R.K., Chrest, F.J., McCoy, M.T., Schneider, E.L., Holbrook, N.J., & Adler, W.H. (1988). Decreased proliferation, interleukin 2 synthesis, and interleukin 2 receptor expression are accompanied by decreased MRNA expression in phytohemagglutinstimulated cells from elderly donors. *J. Clin. Invest. 81*: 1096–1102.

Orr, W.C., & Sohal, R.S. (1992). The effects of catalase gene overexpression on life span and resistance to oxidative stress in transgenic *Drosophila melanogaster*. *Archives Biochem. Biophysics. 297*: 35–41.

Peltomaki, P., Aaltonen, L.A., Sistonen, P., Pylkkanen, L., Mecklin, J.-

P., et al. (1993). Genetic mapping of a locus predisposing to human colorectal cancer. *Science 260*: 810–812.

Rabinowich, H., Goses, Y., Reshef, T. & Klaiman, A. (1985). Interleukin–2 production and activity in aged humans. *Mech. Ageing Dev. 32*: 213–216.

Reveillaud, I., Niedzwiecki, A., Bensch, K.G., & Fleming, J.E. (1991). Expression of bovine superoxide dismutase in *Drosophila melanogaster* augments resistance to oxidative stress. *Mol. Cell. Biol. 11*: 632–640.

Riabowol, K.T., Mizzen, L.A., & Welch, W.J. (1988). Heat shock is lethal to fibroblasts microinjected with antibodies against HSP70. *Science 242*: 433–436.

Riordan, J., Rommens, J.M., Kerem, B.-S., et al. (1989). Identification of the cystic fibrosis gene: cloning and characterization of the complementary CDNA. *Science 245*: 1066–1073.

Rosen, D.R., Siddique, T., Patterson, D., Figlewicz, D.A., Sapp, P., et al. (1993). Mutations in Cu/Zn superoxide dismutase gene are associated with familial amyotrophic lateral sclerosis. *Nature 362*: 59–62.

Rosenberg, S.A. (1992a). The immunotherapy and gene therapy of cancer. *J. Clin. Oncol. 10*: 180–199.

Rosenberg, S.A. (1992b). Gene therapy for cancer. *J. Amer. Med. Assoc. 268*: 2416–2419.

Song, L., Kim, Y.H., Chopra, R.K., Proust, J.J., Nagel, J.E., Nordin, A.A., & Adler, W.H. (1993). Age-related defects in T cell activation and proliferation. *Exp. Gerontol.* In press.

St. George-Hyslop, P., Haines, J., Rogaev, E., Mortilla, M., Vaula, G., et al. (1992). Genetic evidence for a novel familial Alzheimer's disease locus on chromosome 14. *Nature genetics 2*: 330–334.

Stevens, J.G. (1989). Human herpesviruses: A consideration of the latent state. *Microbiol. Rev. 53*: 318–322.

Tanzi, R. E., Vaula, G., Romano, D.M., et al. (1992). Assessment of amyloid B-protein precursor gene mutations in a large set of familial and sporadic Alzheimer disease cases. *Am. J. Hum. Genetics 51*: 273–282.

Thoman, M.L., & Weigle, W.O. (1985). Reconstitution of *in vivo* cell-mediated lympholysis responses in aged mice by interleukin–2. *J. Immunol. 134*: 949–952.

Udelsman, R., Blake, M.J., Stagg, C.A., Li, D., Putney, D.J., & Holbrook, N.J. (1993). Vascular heat shock protein expression in response to stress: endocrine and autonomic regulation of this age-dependent response. *J. Clin. Invest. 91*: 465–473.

Udelsman, R., Blake, M.J., & Holbrook, N.J. (1991). The molecular response to surgical stress: specific and simultaneous heat shock protein induction in the adrenal cortex, aorta, and vena cava. *Surgery I 10*: I 1 25–113 1.

Van Broeckhoven, C., Backhovens, H., Cruts, M., De Winter, G., Bruyland, M., et al. (1992). Mapping of a gene predisposing to early-onset Alzheimer's disease to chromosome 14q24.3. *Nature genetics 2*: 335–339.

Warner, H.R. (1992). Overview: Mechanisms of antioxidant action on life span. In: Antioxidants: Chemical, Physiological, Nutritional and Toxicological Aspects. H. Sies, J. Erdman, Jr., G. Baker III, C. Henry, & G. Williams, eds. Princeton Scientific Publishing Co., Inc. Princeton, N. J.: Princeton Scientific Publishing Co. Inc.

Wasco, W., Brook, J.D., & Tanzi, R.E. (1993). The amyloid precursor-like protein (APLP)gene maps to the long arm of human chromosome 19. *Genomics, 15*: 237–239.

Wispe, J.R., Warner, B.B., Clark, J.C., Dey, C.R., Neuman, J., Glasser, S.W., Crapo, J.D., Chang, L.Y., & Whitsett, J.A. (1992). Human Mn-superoxide dismutase in pulmonary epithelial cells of transgenic mice confers protection from oxygen injury. *J. Biol. Chem. 267*: 23937–23941.

Wolfe, J.H., Deshmane, S.L., & Fraser, N.W. (1992). Herpesvirus vector gene transfer and expression of 6-glucuronidase in the central nervous system of MPS VII mice. *Nature genetics 1*: 379–384.

Understanding and Manipulating the Aging Process Through Transgenic Technology

9

Jon W. Gordon

INTRODUCTION

The 20th century has seen a dramatic increase in the allocation of intellectual and financial resources to basic and applied research. Resulting advances in the physical and biological sciences, in conjunction with improvements in technology that have provided powerful new hardware to investigators, have established "science" as a dominant process by which complex problems are approached. Indeed, the fact that new technological tools are themselves the products of research has further strengthened the influence of scientific method upon modern thinking. As a consequence of these changes, we have come to take for granted the notion that science can solve any problem that exists outside the realm of philosophy.

In this atmosphere of self-confidence, it is somewhat humiliating to acknowledge that our understanding of aging, one of the most profoundly important of all biological processes, is still severely limited. Four features of aging (Strehler, 1982), eloquently discussed by Hayflick (1987), are that it is intrinsic, progressive, deleterious, and universal. Yet, while enumeration of these characteristics assists in defining aging, it does not explain the phenomenon. We are intrigued by the observation that patterns of aging and senescence differ greatly between species, such that in some fishes and insects, developmentally programmed, precipitous demise occurs, while in others, aging, as it is currently understood, does not appear to take place at all. But we intuitively realize that it is not instructive as to the true mechanism(s) of aging in humans. Even objective measures of functional decline (e.g., cardiac output, serum creatinine) fall short of simple visual inspection as a means of assessing the state of aging of an individual. Also unresolved is the simple question of whether aging takes place throughout the life cycle, or only after adulthood is reached. Thus we remain almost totally ignorant of a process which will impact immeasurably upon the character of our lives and ultimately remove us from this planet.

It is our contention that any effort to formally analyze aging will be afflicted with the complication that the process is not separable from external forces. As physical forces act upon the organism, which is a dynamic, adaptable "package" of gene products, it responds by changing its program of gene function. The responses may in some circumstances delay the appearance of stigmata of aging, but in other cases, may hasten it. Thus, while the final result, aging, is correctly regarded as intrinsic, there are extrinsic influences that are difficult to characterize or quantify. For these reasons it is my view that a complete and formal understanding of aging will remain elusive.

This being the case, it is gratifying to turn to the far more practical goal of defining strategies for delaying aging-related dysfunction. Progressive functional decline that occurs with age ultimately manifests as disease, and disease processes can certainly be defined and modified. Attainment of this more pragmatic objective also carries with it the potential for alleviating the devastating social and economic impact of aging-related illness in a rapidly expanding population of elderly people.

Although degenerative diseases associated with aging pose a challenge to medical research, advances in molecular biology provide new approaches to their treatment, and perhaps even their prevention. The most promising new applications of molecular biology are recombinant DNA technology and gene transfer. Because natural selection requires only that the organism live long enough to rear its own young to reproductive age, the developmental program of gene regulation may not be ideal for confronting the changes that occur with advanced age. However, with gene transfer it may well be possible to modify gene regulation in specific tissues of aged individuals so as to forestall the pathological consequences of aging-related changes.

Gene transfer is a newly emerging technology, and much of its use in humans is still in is planning stages. However in animals, experiments have demonstrated the enormous potential of gene, or DNA, therapy for treatment and prevention of disease. The most powerful animal models for experiments in gene therapy are those in which new genetic material is inserted into the germ line. With germ line gene insertion, or "transgenic" technology (Gordon et al., 1980; Gordon & Ruddle, 1981), new genes are permanently incorporated into every cell of the organism and are passed to progeny as Mendelian traits. Thus the problems of efficiency of gene insertion and stability of expression are circumvented.

In this chapter, work ongoing in our laboratory to develop transgenic models for delaying aging-related dysfunction due to cancer will be described (see p. 175). However, to present a single example of the use of transgenic animals in aging research would not do justice to this powerful methodology (for reviews of transgenic research, see Palmiter and Brinster, 1986; Gordon, 1989). Accordingly, I will first review two examples from the extant literature on transgenic technology in aging experiments. These examples include transgenic models of atherosclerosis, and the use of transgenics to investigate the role of oxygen free radicals in aging. In order to provide a suitable background for this discussion as well as presentation of our own data, development of the available methods of gene insertion, the special features of each approach, and the characteristics of foreign gene regulation in transgenic animals, will be briefly described.

DEVELOPMENT OF TRANSGENIC TECHNOLOGY

The first successful production of genetically transformed mice was reported by Gordon et al. (1980). They microinjected the Herpes tk gene into pronuclei of one-celled mouse embryos, implanted the surviving embryos into pseudopregnant foster mice, and examined the DNA of resultant progeny by Southern hybridization for retention of DNA homologous to the microinjected recombinant plasmid. In 3 of 78 mice, clear hybridization to the plasmid material was detected (Gordon et al., 1980). This group (Gordon & Ruddle, 1981) and others (Costantini & Lacy, 1981; Brinster et al., 1981) subsequently noted integration and germ line transmission of the microinjected material. Gordon and Ruddle (1981) termed these transformed mice "transgenic," and thus transgenic technology began.

Although microinjection of pronuclei is still by far the most widely used method for making transgenic mice, two other approaches, each with important unique characteristics, are also employed. The first is retroviral infection. While this technique is not widely used for germ line genetic transformation, it is important for somatic gene therapy.

The second alternative method of gene insertion is embryonic stem (ES) cell mediated gene transfer. Transmission of ES derivatives through the germ line yields offspring bearing the genetic characteristics introduced when the ES cells were cultured. Of the many uses of ES cell mediated gene transfer, the most important is targeted mutagenesis. The ES cell system has unique attributes, and some potential applications of this technology to aging research will be described below.

GENE EXPRESSION IN TRANSGENIC ANIMALS

Before discussing some of the uses of transgenic technology for aging research, it is important to briefly review what has been learned about gene regulation from transgenic animals, and how this knowledge can be applied to studies of mammalian developmental genetics, a discipline which encompasses the aging phase of the life cycle. It is intuitively obvious that three major factors can influence the spatial and temporal pattern of gene expression: *cis*-acting elements which lie close to or within genes, *trans*-acting factors elaborated by differentiated cells that are able to recognize specific gene sequences or accessible regions of chromatin, and the chromosomal environment in which a gene resides. Transgenic animals have proven enormously useful for determining the relative importance of these factors, and the findings have facilitated further development of the technology itself.

Cis-Acting Elements

It was Brinster et al. (1981) who first demonstrated the importance of cis-acting elements to gene regulation. They linked the promoter region of the mouse metallothionein–1 (MT–1) gene to the HSV tk coding sequence and produced transgenic mice. Although ubiquitously expressed, MT–1 is active predominantly in liver and kidney, and is inducible by heavy metals. Brinster et al. (1981) found HSV TK protein primarily in liver and kidney. Moreover, expression in these sites was inducible by cadmium administration. These findings show that tissue specificity of gene expression is determined primarily by cis-acting elements within genes or in their immediate environs. This observation has major implications for use of transgenic technology to target gene expression to specific sites in the genome. For example, linkage of the human growth hormone (hGH) gene to the MT–1 promoter and production of transgenic mice results in animals with very high levels of hGH expression from liver, increased somatic growth, and negative feedback against release of growth hormone from the mouse pituitary (Palmiter et al., 1983). Another important consequence of this regulatory mechanism is that genomic sequences cloned from one species with their cis-acting elements intact are likely to be expressed appropriately when inserted into transgenic animals.

Trans-acting Factors

Trans-acting regulators of gene expression presumably interact with DNA to stimulate transcription of specific genes. These factors can differ in their regulation between species, and such differences can produce aberrant patterns of "transgene" expression. In general, genes inserted across species lines are appropriately expressed; however, interspecies differences in trans-activator production can occasionally yield aberrant expression patterns.

Chromosomal Integration Site

Because even donor gene constructs with strong enhancers can be found to integrate in sites where expression is absent, we may infer that some chromosomal sites are not permissive for expression. In addition, some sites allow expression in tissues where a given transgene is normally not expressed (Leder et al., 1986). However, when the full complement of promoter/enhancer elements is present, the influence of chromosomal integration site is lessened (Grosveld et al., 1987).

APPLICATIONS OF TRANSGENIC TECHNOLOGY TO AGING RESEARCH

In this section, some examples of the use of transgenic animals to study aging and disorders associated with aging will be described. These investigations exploit the capability to faithfully reproduce patterns of donor gene expression by gene transfer, to direct gene expression to specific tissues, and to target mutations in ES cells.

Transgenic Models of Atherosclerosis

Atherosclerosis is an aging-related degenerative process with enormous impact upon health in the elderly. The propensity for developing atherosclerotic lesions is clearly related to the mechanism of lipid transport in blood. Apolipoproteins of various classes complex with lipids and cholesterol and transport them to cells for uptake. Alterations in the apolipoprotein profile can clearly predispose to, or protect against, atherosclerosis.

The low density lipoprotein (LDL) receptor functions to clear LDLs from the blood. High levels of LDL predispose to atherosclerosis. Hofmann et al. (1988) produced transgenic mice carrying the human LDL receptor cDNA under control of the MT–1 promoter. When cadmium was administered to transgenics to stimulate the MT–1 promoter, LDL was cleared from the blood about 10 times more rapidly than in nontransgenic controls. Moreover, the profile of apolipoproteins in plasma was changed, with Apo-E and Apo B–100 reduced by more than 90%. These experiments demonstrate that altered expression of the LDL receptor can significantly modify the lipid profile in plasma, suggesting that genetic engineering of the lipid transport system might be used in the future to delay development of atherosclerosis and its pathological consequences.

The apolipoprotein Apo A-I is present within high density lipoprotein particles (HDLs), high levels of which are associated with reduced risk of atherosclerosis. High level expression of human Apo A-I in transgenic mice raises HDLs and alters their size profile to resemble that found in human plasma (Walsh & Breslow, 1989; Rubin et al., 1991a). When C57BL/6 mice, which manifest reduced HDLs and increased atherogenesis in response to an atherogenic diet, are provided with the human Apo A-I transgene, some inhibition of atherogenesis is found (Rubin et al., 1991b). These findings show that transgenic technology can alter the lipid profile of mice, and might be used to create models for genetic engineering of resistance to atherosclerosis. Experiments with a similar rationale have been extended to the Apo E gene as well. Expression of human Apo E in transgenic mice reduces all plasma lipoproteins except HDL (Shimano et al. 1992).

Plump et al. (1992) have exploited and extended these findings to create a potential mouse model for atherogenic disease. They employed targeted mutagenesis in ES cells to mutate the murine Apo E gene. Homozygous Apo E deficient mice showed 8-fold increases in plasma cholesterol levels when fed a normal diet, while a high fat diet raised cholesterol levels by a factor of 30. These genetically engineered mice also exhibited signs of early atherogenesis. Thus, while this approach does not constitute a model for delayed dysfunction with aging, the accelerated disease in these animals can allow for development of new strategies for hindering the progress of atherosclerotic disease.

Transgenic Models of Altered Oxygen Free Radical Scavenging

One theory of aging that has received much recent attention is the oxygen free radical, or "free radical" theory of aging. This postulates that oxygen free radicals and their derivatives can damage cellular macromolecules, and that such damage eventually leads to a decline in function and/or the appearance of overt pathology (Harman, 1981; 1987). Because of their ubiquitous presence and reactive nature, free radicals have been implicated in a variety of aging-related diseases including cancer, atherosclerosis, diabetes, emphysema, arthritis, post-ischemic reperfusion injury, cirrhosis, and cataracts (Pryor, 1987). Free radicals are generated in a variety of indispensable reactions, but can also result from direct action of oxygen upon organic compounds, or from ionizing radiation (Harman, 1987).

Mammals have developed a free radical scavenging system to defend against this damage. The basic enzymatic pathways begins with production of hydrogen peroxide by superoxide dismutase. There exist two forms of SOD: the mitochondrial enzyme (MnSOD) and the cytoplasmic (Cu/Zn SOD, or SOD–1). Breakdown of H_2O_2 is then accomplished by glutathione peroxidase or catalase (Halliwell et al., 1989). The action of these latter two enzymes generates the highly reactive and damaging hydroxyl radical (Groner et al., 1986). In addition, there is recent evidence that SOD can act directly upon H_2O_2 to produce the hydroxyl radical (Yim et al., 1990). Thus, over-expression of SOD might be predicted to be either beneficial or harmful, depending on the activity of the system for breaking down H_2O_2. In circumstances where SOD activity is limiting and a relative abundance of the oxygen free radical exists, elevation of this enzyme might alleviate free radical damage. However, under conditions where a surfeit of SOD exists, further increases in activity could increase hydroxyl radical production and cause damage. Although it is logical to assume that SOD levels in the organism have been optimized through natural selection, it also must be recognized that natural selection does not exert pressure for optimization of enzyme function in aging. Thus, while it might be expected that global increases in SOD activity throughout development would be detrimental, some tissues of older animals might be expected to be spared from free radical damage by increased activity of SOD.

Indirect evidence that SOD may be important in aging in mammals comes from several sources. Administration of anti-oxidant compounds to mice can increase lifespan by 30% (Harman, 1981), and there is a direct correlation between the ratio of SOD levels to metabolic rates and longevity in mammals (Harman, 1981). A substantial body of data put forward primarily by Groner and his colleagues indicates that overexpression of SOD–1 is responsible for some or all of the neuropathological effects of Down syndrome, a condition that exhibits features of precocious CNS aging and which is frequently accompanied by triplication of the SOD–1 locus. Another fascinating recent observation is that the neurodegenerative disease amyotrophic lateral sclerosis (ALS) is linked to mutations in the SOD–1 gene (Rosen et al., 1993). Apparently, autosomal dominant forms of the disease are tightly linked to mutations found in either axons 2 or 4, usually in highly conserved regions of the molecule. It is presently unclear whether these mutations lead to functional increases or diminutions of enzyme activity (Rosen et al., 1993).

Transgenic technology has great potential for further exploring the role of oxygen free radicals in aging, especially in the CNS. Although the SOD–1 gene has not yet been targeted to specific tissues, such experiments, if conducted on inbred genetic backgrounds, could be highly informative. For example, targeting of gene expression to heart or brain, sites exposed to high levels of free radicals, with studies of lifespan and ischemic damage with age, would be very valuable. Moreover, it is possible to use transgenic technology to determine, very sensitively, whether alterations in the free radical scavenging pathway result in increased or decreased damage to DNA in the tissues where expression is modified. Detection of mutations has been made far more reliable by the development of transgenes which carry genetic markers that can be cloned from the animal, propagated in bacteria, and screened for mutations by a simple colorimetric assay (Vijg & Uitterlinden, 1987). Compound transgenic mice with altered SOD activity could be studied both for longevity and for mutation accumulation in the tissues of interest. Finally, it should be possible to target the SOD–1 locus for mutation, thereby to reduce or eliminate SOD–1, or to replace the enzyme with one of the mutant forms associated with ALS. We have recently cloned the mouse gene for SOD–1 (Benedetto et al., 1991), and we are currently performing targeted mutagenesis in ES cells. Thus, transgenic technology affords new opportunities for penetrating investigations of the role of oxygen free radicals in aging and aging-related disease.

DELAYED DYSFUNCTION IN AGING IN A TRANSGENIC MODEL: CONDITIONAL ABLATION OF CANCER

Attention is now focused on a specific example of a strategy, under investigation in our laboratory, for delaying aging-related dysfunction due to malignant disease.

The approach is based upon recent findings that the Herpes virus thymidine kinase gene, by virtue of its broad substrate specificity, can phosphorylate guanosine analogs such as gancyclovir (GCV), which do not serve as substrates for mammalian TK. Subsequent phosphorylation to triphosphates by mammalian enzymes leads to incorporation of the anaolgs into DNA with resultant inhibition of DNA synthesis. Thus, expression of the HSV tk gene render mammalian cells sensitive to killing by these guanosine analogs. The widest use of this system is for targeted mutagenesis. Exclusion of the tk gene from a donor DNA fragment after homologous recombination with a host sequence can render cells resistant to GCV. Cells with an illegitimate integration event usually retain the tk gene. When searching for homologous recombination these latter transformants can be eliminated from screening by GCV exposure (Capecchi, 1980).

This so-called "TK ablation" has also been used *in vivo* in transgenic animals. Borelli et al. (1989) linked the tk gene to the growth hormone promoter, and were able to ablate somatotropic cells from animals by TK ablation, and Heyman et al. (1989) were able to obtain inducible ablation of lymphoid cells by construction of transgenic mice with a tk gene driven by the immunoglobulin heavy chain enhancer and kappa light chain promoter. The system has also been applied to tumor therapy. When mice with the tk gene expressed in lymphoid cells were induced to form lymphomas by exposure to Abelson virus, successful control of the tumors was accomplished by GCV treatment (Moolten et al., 1990).

Perhaps the most exciting application of TK ablation is described by Culver et al. (1992), who introduced recombinant retroviruses expressing HSV TK into mouse fibroblasts and then inserted the fibroblasts stereotaxically into brain tumors of rats. After GCV administration, profound regression of the brain tumors was noted. Apparently, retroviruses produced by the mouse fibroblasts in the rat brain infected neighboring tumor cells. When GCV was administered, the tumor cells, which actively synthesize DNA because of their high mitotic activity, were destroyed as were the mouse fibroblast producer lines which also divide and express HSV TK (Culver et al., 1992). An important feature of this system is that cells must be synthesizing DNA in order for TK ablation to be successful, because the mechanism of cell killing is based upon incorporation of guanosine analogs into DNA. This stricture is actually an advantage, because normal, non-dividing cells around a tumor would be insensitive to GCV even though they might express the tk gene.

Although the previously reported results are very exciting indeed, they all fall short of perfection as models for TK ablation of cancer. In the case of stereotaxic injection of retrovirus producing cell lines, no certainty exists that every tumor cell will be genetically transformed. In the case of the Abelson virus-induced lymphomas, all lymphoma cells were accessible to TK ablation because the mouse, being transgenic for the tk gene, harbored the gene in every cell. However in this model, all normal lymphoid cells are also subject to TK ablation, and immune deficiency can result from GCV treatment (Heyman et al., 1989).

We have sought a strategy for prophylactic DNA therapy with the HSV tk gene that would allow expression only in malignant cells in the event a cancer should arise. Under these circumstances the tumor would be uniquely accessible to TK ablation; all normal cells would be unaffected. We also sought a model in which tumors are exceedingly difficult to treat with standard therapies.

A condition which satisfies most of these prerequisites is hepatocellular carcinoma (HCC). This disease, very common worldwide, is rarely detected before irreversible spread has occurred. Moreover, many HCC's re-express the a-fetoprotein

(AFP) gene, a gene active normally in fetal liver, yolk sac, and intestine, but not in adult tissues.

Murine AFP gene regulation has been studied in detail by Tilghman and her colleagues. Under typical circumstances this gene is down-regulated at the transcriptional level by several thousand fold within a few weeks of birth. The adult counterpart of AFP, albumin, is activated during fetal life and remains highly active in adult liver. Extensive studies of the murine AFP promoter region have identified three potential enhancers within a 7.6 kb fragment that lies 5' to the cap-site (Godbout et al., 1986; Hammer et al., 1987). These enhancers were shown not to be responsible for postnatal repression of AFP, since grafting of these elements onto the albumin gene did not reduce activity of this latter gene in transgenic mice (Camper & Tilghman, 1989). Rather, a separate DNA element acts as a negative regulator of AFP in adult tissues (Vacher & Tilghman, 1990). Repression of AFP was later also shown to be due in part to an unlinked locus, raf, located on chromosome 15, which acts in a post-translational manner to repress AFP in adult tissues (Vacher et al., 1992). Since many of these regulatory features were elucidated using the AFP promoter region linked either to an AFP minigene or to heterologous genes, we reasoned that if the 7.6 kb promoter region were linked to Herpes tk, this latter gene would express in a manner similar to endogenous AFP. Thus, we would predict the gene to be active in fetal liver, inactive in adult liver, but subject to reactivation in response to stimuli similar to those that activate AFP. We were accordingly hopeful that induction of HCC in AFP/tk transgenic mice would lead to expression of the tk gene in the tumor cells, thus rendering those cells susceptible to TK ablation.

With these considerations in mind, we obtained the 7.6 kb SalI-EcoRI fragment of the mouse AFP promoter region that contained all enhancers and repressors of adult expression, kindly provided by Shirley Tilghman of Princeton University. We also obtained the plasmid pMK from Richard Palmiter of the University of Washington, Seattle. This plasmid contains the entire coding sequence of HSV tk, with elements of the mouse MT–1 promoter and 3' untranslated region (Brinster et al., 1981). We then employed the strategy outlined in Figure 9.1 to link the two DNA fragments in a single plasmid, excise the new chimeric AFP/tk gene as a single SalI fragment and inject it to produce 5 lines of transgenic mice as previously described (Gordon et al., 1980).

One of these lines was selected for further analysis. First, expression of the AFP/tk chimeric gene was studied both in fetuses and adults. For studies of fetal expression, pregnant female mice were sacrificed on day 16 of gestation. Fetuses were removed, and the placentas were saved for determination of transgenic status. Fetal livers were excised and evaluated as potential sites of transgene expression. As a negative control for AFP expression, all tissue above the level of the diaphragm was collected. Tissues from individual animals were then subjected to RNA analysis and northern hybridization, using the tk gene or a cDNA for mouse AFP as probes.

Control studies with the AFP probe confirmed high expression in fetal liver, with no detectable expression in negative control tissue. The same pattern was seen for transgene expression, though absolute levels of tk RNA were substantially lower than for endogenous AFP. Control hybridizations with an actin probe confirmed that comparable amounts of RNA were loaded in each gel slot, and further demonstrated that the presence of the expressed transgene had no apparent effect on endogenous AFP expression.

Expression studies in adult transgenics and control littermates gave somewhat different results. For these studies, mice were sacrificed at 45 days of age. Liver, heart skeletal muscle, spleen, brain, and kidney were excised for northern analysis. When these samples were studied with the AFP probe, the expected result was obtained; that is, no AFP expression was detected in any adult tissue. However, when the samples were probed with tk, low expression was seen in adult liver with no expression detected in any extrahepatic sites. These findings showed that the AFP/tk transgene is not as tightly regulated as the endogenous AFP gene, even though it is driven by the same regulator. Expression of tk RNA,

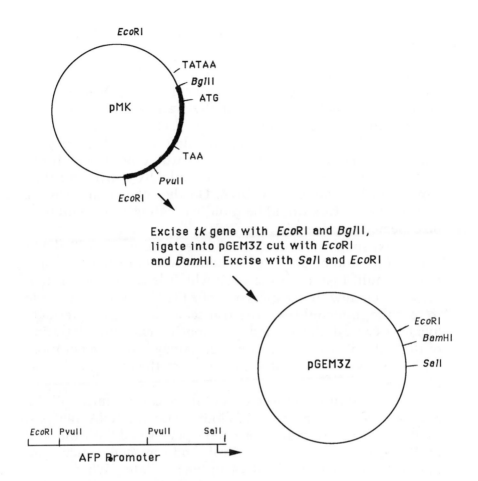

Excise *tk* gene with *EcoRI* and *BglII*,
ligate into pGEM3Z cut with *EcoRI*
and *BamHI*. Excise with *SalI* and *EcoRI*

Ligate *EcoRI:SalI* fragment of AFP promoter to the
SalI:EcoRI fragment of *tk*, and insert into the *EcoRI*
site of pGEM3Z. Excise with *EcoRI* for microinjection.

FIGURE 9.1 Diagram of the cloning strategy for producing the
AFP/HSV tk transgene. In pMK, the thick bar indicates the tk gene.
Note that the endogenous TATA bos is lost during cloning, and the
AFP promoter substitutes for it. The PvuII sites in both fragments
are noted because this enzyme was used to identify transgenic mice.
When PvuII is used, a hybrid restriction fragment containing the 3′
end of the AFP promoter and a substantial portion of the tk gene is
produced. This fragment, which hybridizes both to AFP and tk DNA,
can be used to detect the transgene in mice.

though far lower than AFP in fetuses, is still active in adults, while endogenous AFP is shut down completely. However, despite the residual expression of the transgene in adults, we felt that this transgenic line would be useful for studies of TK ablation of HCC. Our reasoning was that normal hepatocytes, while they might express TK protein, would be insensitive to GCV because they would not be mitotically active and thus would not be synthesizing DNA. On the other hand, cancer cells in these livers would be rapidly dividing and would thus be expected to be sensitive to GCV.

We next sought to determine if, like endogenous AFP, the tk transgene could be activated in adult liver in response to specific stimuli. Insults to the liver which lead to regeneration are associated with re-expression of AFP. The system we chose to test the inducibility of the transgene was carbon tetrachloride (CCl_4) administration. Intraperitoneal administration of this substance causes acute liver damage and regeneration, with expression of AFP 48–72 hours after the insult (Mifflin et al., 1988).

We exposed three transgenic and three control mice to CCL_4 and sacrificed the animals 72 hours later for RNA analysis. When northern hybridizations were performed with the AFP probe, both non-transgenic controls and transgenic mice manifested high levels of AFP RNA in liver isolates. When northern blots were probed with a tk probe, 3/3 transgenic mice expressed the gene at significantly higher levels than transgenic mice treated with placebo. Thus we concluded that the transgene was regulated in much the same manner as endogenous AFP, though peak levels of expression were lower, and re-expression of the gene in adult tissue subjected to chemical injury was less pronounced than observed for the endogenous AFP gene. Nonetheless, because regulation of the tk transgene was very similar to AFP and because transgene RNA was clearly detectable by northern blotting of total RNA, we had reason to be hopeful that this transgenic mouse line would provide a suitable test of TK ablation of HCC. Accordingly, this line was expanded for studies of liver cancer ablation.

A highly suitable model for testing TK ablation in this setting is the chemically induced mouse HCC. After administering dinitrosoethylamine (DEN) in a single neonatal intraperitoneal injection, abnormal groups of cells can be seen throughout the liver at about 20 weeks of age with numerous cancerous nodules appearing at about 30 weeks (Vesselinovitch et al., 1978; Liao et al., 1989). These cancers express high quantities of AFP, and exhibit a pattern of growth and metastatic spread typical of HCC in humans, with pulmonary metastases constituting a prominent manifestation of advanced disease. This model is cumbersome, however, in that a substantial amount of time must elapse between DEN exposure and the onset of the tumor.

In order to obtain a more timely assessment of the potential of TK ablation as prophylaxis for HCC, we chose a transgenic mouse model which develops HCC at an early age. This latter model results from the targeted expression of a potent oncogene, the SV40 T-antigen, to the liver by use of the albumin promoter/enhancer. Albumin is produced in large quantities from adult liver. When the SV40 T-antigen is targeted to liver under albumin regulation, animals express high quantities of the oncogene throughout the liver and rapidly develop dysplastic nodules, many of which ultimately develop into malignant foci (Sandgren et al., 1989; Hino et al., 1991). In their studies, Hino et al. (1991) found cytomegalic changes and high mitotic activity in transgenic livers by 3 to 7 weeks of postnatal life. At 11 weeks frank carcinomas were apparent. By 20 weeks the animals had advanced disease with some pulmonary metastases noted, and died by 7 months of liver failure.

We have studied this model in our own laboratory and found that, at least in our substrain, the disease progresses more rapidly, with adenomatous nodules noted at 2 months of age. In our hands no Albumin/SV40 T-antigen transgenic mouse has lived beyond 4 months. Mice occasionally suffer catastrophic deaths at young ages, and at necropsy are found to have small numbers of very large tumor nodules. We presume the deaths in these instances to be due to vascular obstruction or similar complications of a large, space-occupying lesion. Thus the SV40 T-antigen, when expressed in all hepatocytes as a result of its inheritance through the germ line, dramatically alters liver function and differentiation shortly after birth and kills animals with multifocal carcinomas, and perhaps liver failure as well, by 3–7 months. It is important to note that this disease pattern is not typical hepatocellular cancer, which presumably arises from a single transformed cell. In this model, all cells express the T-antigen and successful treatment of cancerous foci can only be followed by appearance of new malignant lesions. Moreover, de-differentiation of hepatocytes occurs in this model prior to and concomitant with appearance of frank carcinomas, and liver failure is an important component of the disease (Hino et al., 1991). We therefore would expect TK ablation to fail to achieve a cure in these animals. Nonetheless, the model did provide an opportunity to obtain a timely assessment of the potential for this form of gene therapy, and thus we obtained the Albumin/T-antigen transgenics from Dr. N. Tavoloni of the Mount Sinai Deptartment of Neoplastic Diseases, New York, who had himself received them from the laboratory of E.P. Sandgren.

Since some HCC's do not express AFP, our first goal was to determine if the T-antigen model of this disease was associated with AFP transcriptional activation. Albumin/SV40 T-antigen mice were sacrificed for RNA analysis when abdominal enlargement clearly indicated the presence of HCC. Upon sacrifice, large tumor nodules were clearly evident. RNA samples from these livers were subjected to northern analysis using the AFP probe, and were found to express noticeable quantities of AFP, even though the absolute amounts of AFP RNA were far lower than in fetal liver. Nonetheless, the model seemed suitable for testing the TK ablation strategy. We therefore crossed our hemizygous AFP/tk transgenics with the albumin/SV40 T-antigen animals to generate progeny of four different genotypes: negative animals, animals positive for the tk transgene only, animals with the SV40 T-antigen transgene only, and compound transgenic animals which carried both transgenes.

It is in this latter group that we sought to determine the efficacy of GCV therapy. The other mice served as important controls. Mice with the SV40 T-antigen only were used to follow the development of HCC with and without GCV therapy. These animals were expected to develop HCC and expire at an early age whether treated with GCV or placebo (saline). These animals thus served as standards for establishing the aggressiveness of untreated HCC in our subline of mice, and were also used to factor out non-specific anti-tumorigenic, or tumor promoting, effects of GCV. Mice with the tk transgene only were also important to demonstrate that GCV treatment in the absence of HCC was not toxic. In addition, measurement of the lifespans of these animals when treated either with GCV or placebo was considered necessary for ruling out non-specific effects of transgene integration and expression. It was also necessary to treat some of the compound transgenics with saline to rule out the possibility that TK production would alter the course of SV40 T-antigen induced HCC. Therefore all four groups of animals were divided into GCV and placebo treatment groups. The general strategy for ablating HCC's in the compound transgenics was to administer GCV in an early phase of the disease in order that massive tumor lysis not pose an independent threat to survival. Parameters followed during treatment included longevity, liver weight as a percentage of total body weight, and changes in expression of the tk transgene in tumors that might appear despite treatment with GCV. Results to be presented here will be confined to longevity, which can be taken as an indirect measure of the delay of dysfunction due to tumor growth.

Turning first to the various control groups, the following findings were noteworthy. GCV administration appeared not to be toxic to mice with the AFP/tk transgene only. This finding confirmed our expectation that GCV would not be toxic in the absence of cell mitosis, even if the tk gene was active. SV40 T-antigen transgenics and compound transgenics had indistinguishable patterns of HCC development and associated pathology. Thus, the presence and expression of the Herpes protein did not affect the course of liver disease. Mice with the T-antigen transgene only, whether given GCV or placebo, exhibited the same time course of HCC development. Thus, GCV had not obvious non-specific antitumor effect. Compound transgenics given placebo were also very similar to mice with the T-antigen alone given either placebo or GCV, results which show that TK production did not affect the action of the T-antigen upon the liver. All mice without the T-antigen gene, whether given placebo or GCV, had no discernible pathology.

In the first experimental group given GCV, compound transgenics survived significantly longer than those given placebo. In animals given placebo, the longest survival time was 126 days, while in treatment group 1, five compound transgenics lived more than 149 days whereupon GCV treatment was stopped. Perhaps most striking was the difference in abdominal enlargement between GCV and control mice. In controls, significant enlargement was always observed within 3 months of birth, while such enlargement was remarkably delayed in the GCV treatment group. This observation is illustrated in Figure 9.2 for two compound transgenics of treatment group 2, aged 120 days. One of these animals was given GCV, the other placebo. As shown, profound abdominal enlargement is manifest in the animal given placebo, while the mouse receiving GCV is normal in appearance. In fact, mice from group 1 treated with GCV often expired with little or no noticeable abdominal enlargement. Several of these animals were found to be profoundly anemic at the time of death. We interpret these findings as indicating the cause of death to be liver failure rather than HCC. Several sudden deaths were seen in relatively young compound transgenics given saline or mice with the SV40 T-antigen gene only, with or without GCV treatment. Upon sacrifice these animals were found to have one or more large tumor nodules.

In mice given GCV according to a second, higher dose regimen, more effective delay of tumor development was observed. Several of these animals are still alive at an age exceeding 150 days, and they manifest no noticeable pathology. In one animal, GCV treatment was stopped at 140 days. This

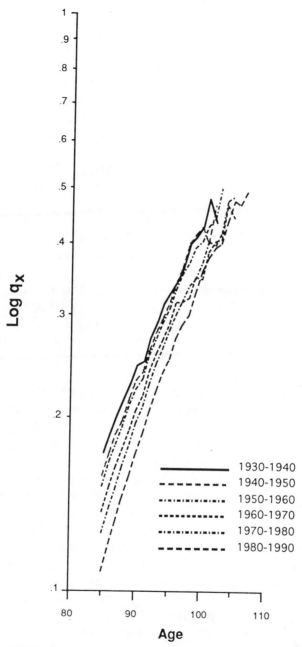

FIGURE 10.7 The mortality rates at advanced ages in England and
Wales, plotted as natural log of mortality per year against age.
(Replotted from data of Thatcher, 1992.)

mouse has gradually experienced abdominal enlargement, indicative that cessation of GCV therapy is allowing tumor growth. In several other animals, continuation of GCV therapy has maintained these animals in apparent good health.

A striking further observation was made on a compound transgenic animal from group 2 that received GCV and that is now approximately 140 days old. This animal was subjected to liver biopsy in order to evaluate T-antigen, AFP, and tk gene expression. When the liver was examined at the time of biopsy, only a single region of dysplasia approximately 3 mm in diameter was seen. Thus, this animal is essentially disease-free. This finding contrasts dramatically with placebo-treated animals or even group 1 compound transgenics treated with GCV. In these other animals, several prominent tumor nodules were always present at the time of death. These results suggest that optimization of TK ablation protocols can profoundly affect results. Moreover, successful treatment in group 2 indicates that even the most aggressive cancers might be effectively controlled by TK ablation after appropriate prophylactic DNA therapy.

In addition to the demonstrable efficacy of TK ablation for AFP-expressing liver cancers, the present studies offer new opportunities for basic studies of the evolution of malignant disease. Many patients treated for cancer with standard chemotherapy or radiation suffer recurrences that manifest as metastases. When a new round of therapy is undertaken, the recurrent malignancies are more difficult to treat than the original tumor. The mechanism(s) by which tumors become refractory to therapy are rarely understood clearly, but they may well result from genetic changes within the tumor cells. Tumor cells which must establish metastatic foci in environments that are quite different from that in which the progenitor cancer cell arose may be subject to selective pressure that leads to emergence of a genetic heterogeneity. Such heterogeneity might not only favor survival of metastatic foci, it might also render the tumor more resistant to antineoplastic agents. In most settings it is difficult to determine the genetic factors that might lead to improved tumor survival, but in our transgenic mice the genes involved are easily pinpointed: they are the AFP and HSV tk genes. If tumors recur in our animals during GCV treatment, we must infer that TK ablation is no longer effective and thus, that the cell has altered regulation at one of these 2 loci such that TK is no longer produced. Thus our animals offer us the opportunity to determine if gene deletion, rearrangement, or altered regulation at these loci is responsible for tumor recurrence. Our findings may well provide clues to the mechanism(s) by which human cancers survive therapy, acquire resistance to treatment, and metastasize.

It should be re-emphasized that the tumor model studied here would be expected to be far more refractory to treatment than a typical malignancy, which exists as a single clone of cancer cells within large field of non-malignant tissue. This situation is better approximated by the DEN model for HCC, studies of which are ongoing in our laboratory. This realization gives us a high degree of confidence that refined DNA therapy, if performed according to a similar strategy as that employed here, could significantly delay dysfunction due to one of the most common conditions of aging, cancer. It is also noteworthy that GCV treatment is essentially non-toxic and that thus what are now some of the most serious and debilitating diseases might in the future be treated outside of the hospital setting.

ACKNOWLEDGMENTS

This work was supported in part by NIH grants CA42103 and AI24460. I thank Paola Macri for postdoctoral collaboration in research and manuscript preparation, and Marc Gordon for technical assistance in the research.

REFERENCES

Avraham, K.B., Schickler, M., Sapoznikov, D., Yarom, R., and Groner Y., 1988. Down's syndrome:abnormal neuromuscular junction in tongue of transgenic mice with elevated levels of human Cu/Zn-superoxide dismutase. *Cell 54*: 823–829.

Belayew, A., and Tilghman, S.M., 1982. Genetic analysis of a-fetoprotein synthesis in mice. *Mol. Cell. Biol. 2*: 1427–1435.

Benedetto, M.T., Anzai, Y., and Gordon, J.W., 1991. Isolation and
analysis of the mouse genomic sequence encoding Cu/Zn superoxide dismutase. *Gene 99*: 191–195.

Borrelli, E., Heyman, R., Arias, C., Sawxhenko, P.E., and Evans,
R.M., 1989. Transgenic mice with inducible dwarfism. *Nature
339*: 538–541.

Brinster, R.L., Chen, H.Y., Trumbauer, M.E., Senear, A.W., Warren,
R., and Palmiter, R.D., 1981. Somatic expression of herpes thymidine kinase in mice following injection of a fusion gene into
eggs. *Cell 27*: 223–231.

Camper S.A., and Tilghman, S.M., 1989. Postnatal repression of the
a-fetoprotein gene is enhancer independent. *Genes & Develop.
3*: 537–546.

Capecchi, M.R. 1980. High efficiency transformation by direct microinjection of DNA into cultured mammalian cells. *Cell 22*:
479–488.

Costantini, F., and Lacy, E. 1981. Introduction of a rabbit b-globin
gene into the mouse line. *Nature 294*: 92–94.

Culver, K.W., Ram, Z., Wallbridge, S., Ishii, H., Oldfield, E.H., and
Blaese, R.M., 1992. In vivo gene transfer with retroviral vector-
producer cells for treatment of experimental brain tumors. *Science 256*: 1550–1552.

Elroy-Stein, O., Bernstein, Y., and Groner, Y., 1986. Overproduction
of human Cu/Zn superoxide dismutase in transfected cells: ex-
tenuation of paraquat-mediated cytotoxicity and enhancement
of lipid peroxidation. *EMBO J. 5*: 615–622.

Elroy-Stein, O., and Groner, Y., 1988. Impaired neurotransmitter uptake in PC12 cells overexpressing human Cu/Zn superoxide dismutase—implication of gene dosage effects in Down syndrome. *Cell 52*: 259–267.

Epstein, C.J., Avraham, K.B., Lovett, M., Smith, S., Elroy-Stein, O.,
Rotman, G., Bry, C., and Groner Y., 1987. Transgenic mice increased Cu/Zn-superoxide dismutase activity: Animal model of
dosage effects in Down Syndrome. *Proc. Natl. Acad. Sci. USA
84*: 8044–8048.

Evans, M.J., and Kaufman, M.H. 1981. Establishment in culture of
pluripotential cells from mouse embryos. *Nature 292*: 154–156.

Farrington, J.A., Ebert, M., Land, E.J., and Fletcher, K., 1973. Pulse radiolysis studies of the reaction of paraquat radical with oxygen. Implications for the mode of action of bipyridyl herbicides. *Bioch. Biophys. Acta 314*: 372–381.

Godbout, R., Ingram, R., and Tilghman, S.M., 1986. Multiple regulatory elements in the intergenic region between the a-fetoprotein gene and albumin gene. *Mol. Cell. Biol. 6*: 477–487.

Gordon, J.W. 1989. Transgenic animals. *Int. Rev. Cytol. 115*: 171–230.

Gordon, J.W., Scangos, G.A., Plotkin, D.J., Barbosa, J.A., and Ruddle, F.H. 1980. Genetic transformation of mouse embryos by microinjection of purified DNA. *Proc. Natl. Acad. Sci. USA 77*: 7380–7384.

Gordon, J.W., and Ruddle, F.H. 1981. Integration and stable germ line transmission of genes injected into mouse pronuclei. *Science 214*: 1244–1246.

Graessmann, A., Graessmann, M., Topp, W.C., and Botchan, M. 1979. Retransformation of a simian virus 40 revertant cell line, which is resistant to viral and DNA infections, by microinjection of viral DNA. *J. Virol. 32*: 989–994.

Groner, Y., Elroy-Stein, O., Bernstein, Y., Dafni, N., Levanon, D., Danciger, E., and Neer, A., 1986. Molecular genetics of Down's syndrome: over-expression of transfected human CuZn-superoxide dismutase gene and the consequent physiological changes. *Cold Spr. Harb. Symp. Quant. Biol. LI*: 381–393.

Grosveld, F., van Assendelft G.B., Greaves D.R., and Kollias G., 1987. Position-independent, high-level expression of the human b-globin gene in transgenic mice. *Cell 51*: 975–985.

Halliwell, B., and Gutteridge, J.M.C., 1989. Free Radicals in Biology and Medicine, 2nd Edition, Clarendon, Press, Oxford.

Hammer, R.E., Krumlauf, R., Camper, S.A., Brinster, R.L., and Tilghman, S.M., 1987. Diversity of alpha-fetoprotein gene expression in mice is generated by a combination of separate enhancer elements. *Science 235*: 53–58.

Harman, D., 1981. The aging process. *Proc. Natl. Acad. Sci. USA 78*: 7124–7128.

Harman, D., 1987. The free-radical theory of aging. In: Modern Biological theories of Aging, H.R. Warner, R.N. Butler, R.L. Sprott, and E.L. Schneider, (eds). Raven Press, New York, NY pp. 81–87.

Hassan, H.M., and Fridovich, I., 1979. Intracellular production of superoxide radical and of hydrogen peroxide by redox active compounds. *Arch. Biochem. Biophy. 196*: 385–395.

Heyman, R.A., Borreli, E., Lesley, J., Anderson, D., Richman, D.D.,

Baird, S.M., Hyman, R., and Evans, R.M., 1989. Thymidine kinase obliteration: creation of transgenic mice with controlled immune deficiency. *Proc. Natl. Acad. Sci. USA 84*: 2698–2702.

Hino, O., Kitagawa, T., Nomura, K., Ohtake, K., Cui, L., Furuta, Y., and Aizawa, S., 1991. Hepatocarcinogenesis in transgenic mice carrying albumin-promoted SV40 T antigen gene. *Jpn. J. Cancer Res. 82*: 1226–1233.

Hoffmann, S.L., Russell D.W., Brown M.S., Goldstein J.L., and Hammer R.E., 1988. Overexpression of low density lipoprotein (LDL) receptor eliminates LDL from plasma in transgenic mice. *Science 239*: 1277–1281.

Jaenisch, R., 1976. Germ line integration and Mendelian transmission of the exogenous Moloney leukemia virus. *Proc. Natl. Acad. Sci. USA 73*: 1260–1264.

Jahner, D., Haase, K., Mulligan, R., and Jaenisch R., 1985. Insertion of the bacterial gpt gene into the germ line of mice by retroviral infection. *Proc. Natl. Acad. Sci. USA 82*: 6927–6931.

Krumlauf, R., Hammer, R.E., Tilghman, S.M., and Brinster, R., 1985. Developmental regulation for a-fetoprotein genes in transgenic mice. *Mol. Cell. Biol. 5*: 1639–1648.

Leder, A., Pattengale, P.K., Kuo, A., Stewart, T.A., and Leder, P., 1986. Consequences of widespread deregulation of the c-myc gene in transgenic mice:multiple neoplasms and normal development. *Cell 45*: 485–495.

Leiman-Hurwitz, J., Dafni, N., Lavie, V., and Groner, Y., 1982. Human cytoplasmic superoxide dismutase cDNA clone: a probe for studying the molecular biology of Down's syndrome. *Proc. Natl. Acad. Sci. USA 79*: 2828–2811.

Levanon, D., Lieman-Hurwitz, J., Dafni, N., Wigderson, M., Sherman, L., Bernstein, Y., Laver-Rudich, Z., Danciger, E., Stein, O., and Groner, Y., 1985. Architecture and anatomy of the chromosomal locus in human chromosome encoding the Cu/Zn superoxide dismutase. *EMBO J. 4*: 77–84.

Liao, W.S.L., Ma, K.-T., and Becker, F.F., 1989. Altered expression of acute-phase reactants in mouse liver tumors. *Mol. Carcinogenesis 1*: 260–266.

Mann, J.R., Mulligan, R.C., and Baltimore, D., 1983. Construction of retrovirus packaging mutant and its use to produce helper-free defective retrovirus. *Cell 33*: 153–159.

Mansour, S.L., Thomas, K.R., and Capecchi, M.R., 1988. Disruption of the proto-oncogene int–2 in mouse embryo-derived stem cells: a general strategy for targeting mutations to non-selectable genes. *Nature 336*: 348–352.

Martin, G.R. 1981. Isolation of a pluripotent cell line from early mouse embryos cultured in medium conditioned by teratocarcinoma stem cells. *Proc. Natl. Acad. Sci. USA 78*: 7634–7638.

Mifflin, R.C., Moller P.C., and Papaconstantinou, J., 1988. Genetic analysis of L-ethionine-mediated induction of alpha-fetoprotein in mice. *Somatic Cell Mol. Genet. 14*: 553–566.

Moody, C.S., and Hassan, H.M., 1982. Mutagenicity of oxygen free radicals. *Proc. Natl. Acad. Sci. USA 79*: 2855–2859.

Moolten, F.L., Wells, J.M., Heyman, R.A., and Evans, R.M., 1990. Lymphoma regression induced by ganciclovir in mice bearing a herpes thymidine kinase transgene. *Human gene therapy 1*: 125–134.

Palmiter, R.D., and Brinster, R.L. 1986. Germ-line transformation of mice. *Ann. Rev. Genet. 20*: 465–499.

Palmiter, R.D., Norstedt, G., Gelinas, R.E., Hammer, R.E., and Brinster, R.L., 1983. Metallothionein-human GH genes stimulate growth of mice. *Science 222*: 809–814.

Plump, A.S., Smith, J.D., Hayek, T., Aalta-Setala, K., Walsh, A., Verstuyft, J.G., Rubin, E.M., and Breslow, J.L., 1992. Severe hypercholesterolemia and atherosclerosis in apolipoprotein E-deficient mice created by homologous recombination in ES cells. *Cell 71*: 343–353.

Pryor, W.A. 1987. The free-radical theory of aging revisited: A critique and a suggested disease-specific theory. In: Modern Biological theories of Aging, H.R. Warner, R.N. Butler, R.L. Sprott, and E.L. Schneider, (eds). Raven Press, New York, NY pp. 89–112.

Przedborski, S., Kostic, V., Jackson-Lewis, V., Naini, A.B., Simonetti, S., Fahn, S., Carlson, E., Epstein, C.J., and Cadet, J.L., 1992. Transgenic mice with increased Cu/Zn-superoxide dismutase activity are resistant to N-methyl–4-phenyl–1,2,3,6-tetrahydropyridine-induced neurotoxicity. *J. Neuroscience. 12*: 1658–1667.

Rosen, D.R., Siddique, T., Patterson D., Figlewicz, D.A., Sapp, P., Hentati, A., Donaldson, D., Goto, J., O'Regan, J.P., Deng, H.-X., Ragman, Z., Krizus, A., McKenna-Yasek, D., Cayabykab, A., Gaston, S.M., Berger, R., Tanzi, R.E., Halperin, J.J., Herzfeldt, B., Van den Bergh, R., Hung, W.-Y., Bird, T., Deng, G., Mulder, D.W., Smyth, C., Laing, N.G., Soriano, E., Pericak-Vance, M.A., H aines, J., Rouleau, G.A., Gusella, J.S., Horvitz, H.R., and Brown, R.H., 1993. Mutations in Cu/Zn superoxide dismutase gene are associated with familial amyotrophic lateral sclerosis. *Nature* *362*: 59–62.

Rubin, E.M., Ishida B.Y., Clift S.M., and Krauss, R.M., 1991a. Expression of human apolipoprotein A-I in transgenic mice results in reduced plasma levels of murine apolipoprotein A-I and the appearance of two new high density lipoprotein size subclasses. *Proc. Natl. Acad. Sci. USA 88*: 434–438.

Rubin, E.M., Krauss R.M., Spangeler E.A., Verstuyft J.G., and Clift S.M., 1991b. Inhibition of early atherogenesis in transgenic mice by human apolipoprotein AI. *Nature 353*: 265–267.

Sandgren, E.P., Quaife, C.J., Pinkert, C.A., Palmiter, R.D., and Brinster R.L., 1989. Oncogene-induced liver neoplasia in transgenic mice. *Oncogene 4*: 715–724.

Shimano, H., Yamada, N., Katsuki, M., Shimada, M., Gotoda, T., Harada, K., Murase, T., Fukazawa, C., Takaku, F., and Yazaki, Y., 1992. Overexpression of apolipoprotein E in transgenic mice: Marked reduction in plasma lipoproteins except high density lipoprotein and resistance against diet-induced hypercholesterolemia. *Proc. Natl. Acad. Sci. USA. 89*: 1750–1754.

Smithies, O., Grett, R.G., Boggs, S.S., Koralewski, M.A., and Kucherlapati, R.S., 1985. Insertion of DNA sequences into the human chromosomal b-globin locus by homologous recombination. *Nature 317*: 230–234.

Strehler, B.L. 1982: Ageing: Concepts and theories. In: *Lectures on Gerontology*, edited by A Viidik. Academic Press, New York, pp. 1–57.

Thompson, S., Clarke, A.R., Pow, A.M., Hooper, M.L., and Melton, D.W., 1989. Germ line transmission and expression of corrected HPRT gene produced by gene targeting in embryonic stem cells. *Cell 56*: 313–321.

Vacher, J., Camper, S.A., Krumlauf, R., Compton, R.S., and Tilghman, S.M., 1992. raf regulates the postnatal repression of the mouse a-fetoprotein gene at the posttranscriptional level. *Mol. Cell. Biol. 12*: 856–864.

Vacher, J., and Tilghman, S.M., 1990. Dominant negative regulation of the mouse a-fetoprotein gene in adult liver. *Science 250*: 1732–1735.

van der Putten, H., Botteri, H., Miller, F.M., Rosenfeld, A.D., Fan, M.G., Evans, R.M., and Verma, I. 1985. Efficient insertion of genes into the mouse germ line via retroviral vectors. *Proc. Natl. Acad. Sci. USA 82*: 6148–6152.

Vesselinovitch, S.D., Mihalalovich, N., and Rao, K.V.N., 1978. Morphological and metastatic nature of induced hepatic nodular lesions in C57BL X C3H F1 mice. *Cancer Res. 38*: 2003–2010.

Vijg, J., and Uitterlinden, A.G., 1987. A search for DNA alterations in the aging mammalian genome: an experimental strategy. *Mech. Aging Develop. 41*: 47–63.

Walsh A., Ito Y., and Breslow, J.L., 1989. High levels of human apolipoprotein A-I in transgenic mice result in increased plasma levels of small high density lipoprotein (HDL) particles comparable to human HDL_3. *J. Biol. Chem. 11*: 6488–6494.

Yarom, R., Sapoznikov, D., Havivi, Y., Avraham, K.B., Schickler, M., and Groner, Y., 1988. Premature aging changes in neuromuscular junctions of transgenic mice with an extra human CuZn-SOD gene: a model for tongue pathology in Down's syndrome. *J. Neurological Sci. 88*: 41–53.

Yim, M.B., Chock, P.B., and Stadtamn, E.R., 1990. Copper, zinc superoxide dismutase catalyzes hydroxyl radical production from hydrogen peroxide. *Proc. Natl. Acad. Sci. USA 87*: 5006–5010.

Ziljstra, M., Box, M., Simister, N.E., Loring, J.M., Raulet D.H., and Jaenisch, R., 1990. B_2-microglobulin deficient mice lack CD–8+ cytolytic T cells. *Nature 344*: 742–746.

The Plasticity of Life Histories in Natural Populations of Animals: Insights Into the Modifiability of Human Aging Processes

10

Caleb E. Finch

INTRODUCTION

Human populations vary widely in the patterns of age-related diseases and life expectancy. Animal populations in the natural world also show differences that indicate strong environmental influences during development and throughout life on mortality risks and other outcomes of aging. These variations in life history imply a deep plasticity in life history regulation that arises through variations in gene expression, i.e., at an epigenetic level. These insights support optimism about the modifiability of human aging processes through epigenetic approaches.

Human life spans are always finite. Even if we maintained mortality risks from puberty—the safest age in life, as Simms (1945) showed—onwards, the life expectancy would be increased only to about 1,200 years. Moreover, no one can escape the irreducible fact that, over extended time, mortality risks increase and do so with an acceleration that more-or-less doubles every 8 years in all known human populations (Comfort, 1979; Finch, 1990, pp. 22–23). This outcome of aging might simply be the result of unavoidable exposure to biohazards from the external and internal environment that tend to leave long-lasting effects on our systems.

To begin with, exposure to sunlight and to the myriad natural carcinogens in food and in the atmosphere guarantee some level of damage in our cells, particularly DNA modifications that can increase the risk of cancer. Exposure to circulating sex hormones also furthers the risk of abnormal growths, including cancer, in reproductive tissues. Exposure to fats and glucose furthers the risk of damage to blood vessels and other slowly replaced cells and molecules through glycation, free radical oxidation, and other chemical reactions. Under some circumstances, stress and elevated glucocorticoids can irreversibly damage neurons (see chapter 7). These effects are in many cases slow and insidious, taking decades before ill effects are apparent. Added to these chemoenvironmental insults are hazards from trauma and accidents.

We must also include the numerous hereditary diseases with adult onset, such as the blood lipid disorders and type II diabetes. Dementia, which shows strong familial trends in cases of Alzheimer's disease, will account for even more morbidity at later ages, possibly afflicting 30–50% by the age of 85 years. Alzheimer's disease is at least fivefold more common than the next most common inherited disorder, familial hypercholesteremia (Farrer et al., 1990). Recent surveys of human populations in Boston, Gothenberg (Sweden), and Shanghai show about the same prevalence of dementia after 80 years (see chapter 6).

These global features of human diseases during aging appear to support the traditional conclusion that the human life span is biologically limited (Fries, 1980), say to 120 years, which is about the maximum credible record, held by Shigichio Izumi (Guinness Book of World Records, 1987).

At a cellular level, there are at least two examples of pacemakers. In most mammals, the ovary has a fixed number of oocytes and primary follicles that are lost irreversibly, starting shortly after birth (Fig. 10.1). The exhaustion of ovarian germ cells is complete by midlife and is the cause of menopause (Gosden, 1985; Finch, 1990, pp. 165–166, 493–495). Another widely recognized clock is the finite replicative capacity of cultured human cells. Together, this evidence suggests the gloomy perspective that there are built in clocks of one sort or another that tick off our allotted biological time with an inevitability like the time kept by pulsing stars.

In contrast, I propose a different perspective: *that the human life span potential is not determined by any rigid clock*. My perspective draws from the fundamental plasticity of life histories observed throughout the biological world, in millions of animal and plant species. Examples are given from species, followed by a revisiting of the human condition and prospects for extending the healthy span of life, whatever its length.

EXAMPLES OF PLASTICITY IN SENESCENCE

Evolutionary biologists recognize that the duration of the reproductive schedule is one of the most important regulators of the adult phase, since the adult phase must last long enough for reproduction to maintain the population balance. Otherwise, of course, the species would become extinct. Many of the following examples show that the life span and details of senescence are altered in relation to the reproductive schedule. At one extreme are the species, scattered throughout plants and animals that die soon after their first and only season of reproduction. This type of reproductive schedule is called *semelparous*, to distinguish it from the *iteroparous* schedule of the far more numerous species that reproduce repeatedly.

Semelparity has not been observed in some evolutionary radiations, particularly in amphibia, reptiles, and birds. These species tend to be long-lived (at least five years) and

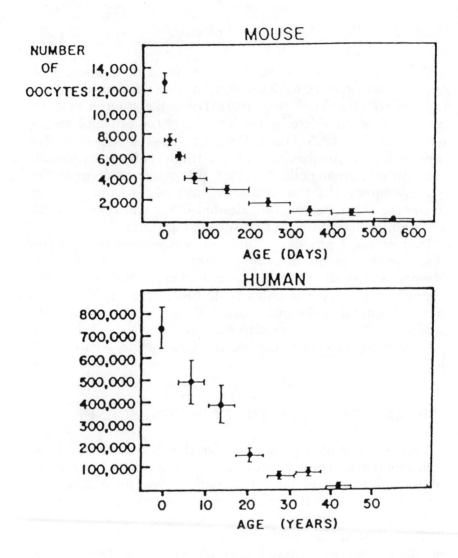

FIGURE 10.1 The ovary has a fixed number of oocytes and primary follicles that are lost irreversibly, starting shortly after birth, with kinetics like the decay of radiosotopes. (*Source*: Finch, 1990, p. 165.)

with unknown upper limits to life span and the duration of fertility (Finch, 1990, pp. 143–150, 221). In particular, many birds show little or no decline in reproduction during long adult life spans. For example, the fulmar, a marine bird which nests in the Orkney Islands north of Scotland, has a reproductive schedule that is very similar to humans. Reproduction can begin by 12–14 years, but the success of parenting does not reach its peak until after 20 years (Fig. 10.2) (Ollason & Dunnett, 1988). Moreover, longitudinal studies have not detected either declines in egg laying or increases in mortality at least into the mid-thirties. Nothing is known about whether oogenesis continues during adult life in these or other birds. Pending more extended study, I conclude provisionally that fulmars and many other vertebrates have a slower kinetics of senescence than in mammals of similar size and overall mortality rates. Having set an upper limit to senescence with this example, the next examples describe the more rapid senescence of semelparous species.

Marsupial Mice

Among mammals, semelparity is best described in ten species of mouse-sized marsupials that live in Australia. In *Antechinus stuartii*, for example, the males die universally after their first and only season of mating (Lee & Cockburn, 1985; Finch, 1990, pp. 95–97; Diamond, 1982). Females, however, typically survive to another season, when a few have a second litter. The death in males is caused by a stress syndrome, with huge elevations of cortisol that, in turn cause suppression of immune function, impaired ingestion of food, GI ulcers, and weight loss. The stress is attributed to mating-related behaviors, including fighting and the prolonged bouts of copulation. In contrast, if male *Antichinus stuartii* are isolated in the lab before breeding starts, then the side-lined males will survive for at least 3 years. Moreover, males of the closely related *A. bilarni* are iteroparous and survive for several years. Thus,

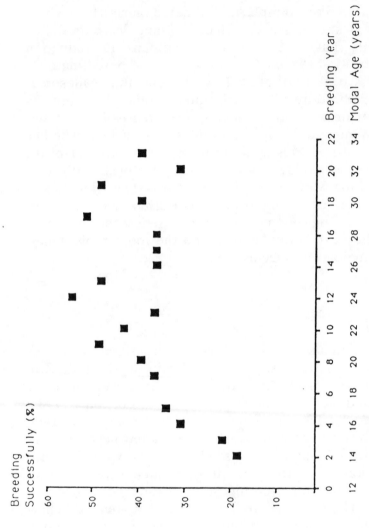

FIGURE 10.2 Fulmars, a marine bird (Fulmarus glacialis), have an extended reproductive schedule that shows no evidence of reproductive decline up through the mid-thirties. The increased success of conjugal pairs in rearing their offspring to fledge may depend on learning about predators, the building of nests, and foraging. (Redrawn from Ollason and Dunnett, 1988.)

the pacemaker for the life span of the semelparous male marsupial mice is environmentally triggered and not intrinsic. Overall, semelparity is rare in mammals.

Ferox Salmon, Pacific Salmon, and American Shad

Fish have maximum life spans in nature that range more than a hundredfold, from the short-lived annual cyprinodonts that succumb to the drying out of their seasonal rain puddles to rockfish, sturgeon, and other iteroparous fish that live a good hundred or more years with few indications of senescence (Finch, 1990, pp. 216–219). Moreover, in many species, the life history is conditional, and can be semelparous or iteroparous. Indeed, the range of fish life histories is remarkable.

For example, brown trout (*Salmo trutta*) have two life history paths with different growth potential and life expectancy (Figure 10.3A). In Scotland and Ireland, fisherman prize the huge ferox trout that grow to more than 30 pounds at ages of at least 20 years (Campbell, 1979; Ferguson & Mason, 1981; Hamilton et al., 1989). Other brown trout in the same waters remain small, with maximum life spans of 4–6 years. Figure 10.3 shows the growth of ferox and ordinary browns which diverges at about 6 years when ferox have a growth spurt. The key appears to be a different diet, since the ferox trout prey on and ingest small fish, while the ordinary small browns are largely particle feeders. Whatever the explanation, learned behavior or genetic polymorphisms, ferox give a strident counter example to the belief that meager diets are the only approach to extended longevity. *Pace*, Roy Walford (Weindruch & Walford, 1988).

A famous example of semelparity is given by the five species of Pacific salmon (*Oncorhynchus*), in which both genders die soon after spawning (Finch, 1990. pp. 83–95; Robertson et al., 1961a,b; Robertson, 1961; Van Dyke & Fobes, 1990), except in the case of a life history variant. Like the male marsupial mice, the Pacific salmon are killed by a stress syndrome with elevated cortisol. Numerous degenerative changes include not only immune suppression, cessation of feeding, and wasting of muscle,

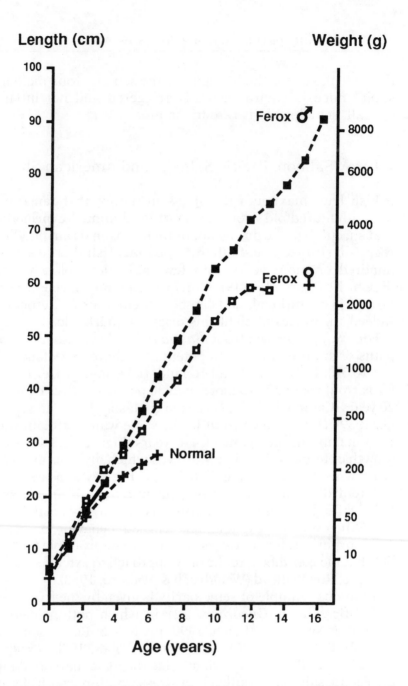

FIGURE 10.3 (A) Life history paths of brown trout. (B) The growth of normal brown trout and ferox, which diverges at about 6 years, when ferox have a growth spurt. (*Source*: Finch, 1990, p. 142.)

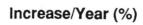

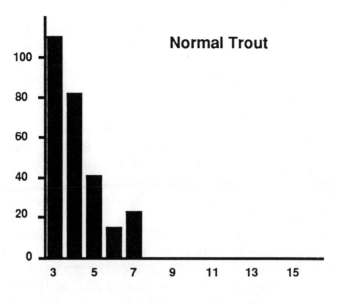

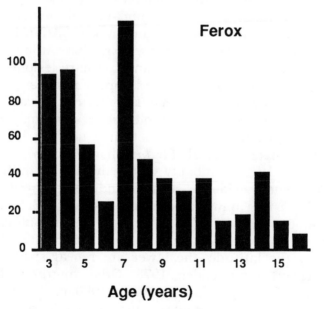

FIGURE 10.3 (*Continued*)

but also coronary artery degeneration with intimal cell proliferation. These changes can be prevented by castration of young
salmon in which case the castrates continue to grow and outlive
their peers by twofold (Robertson, 1961). The pacemaker of
these changes requires maturation or elevations of gonadal steroids (van Overbeeke & McBride, 1971). However, other stresses
associated with reproduction besides the mere act of spawning
alone may be required for death (Fagerlund, 1967). Besides the
strenuous migration upstream, salmon then have further de-
manding activities: males fight for access to ripe females, while
females move stones around in the stream to prepare a nest
(redd) before egg-laying.

In contrast to adults, if juvenile males mature precociously,
some will survive spawning (Robertson, 1957). Here we see an
alternate life history, which increases the reproductive opportunity of the population. A diversity of ages at first reproduction is not uncommon in animals; this type of developmental
plasticity is viewed as "bet-hedging" in evolutionary biology.

Precocious maturation is common in Atlantic salmon
(*Salmo*), which generally survive spawning. Atlantic salmon
also have elevations of cortisol and coronary lesions that persist through successive years and appear to become more severe (Saunders & Farrell, 1988). Long-term survival in nature
despite progressive gross pathological lesions may be more
common than realized and is certainly not restricted to humans. The greater survival of *Salmo* than *Oncorhynchus* is a recently derived trait, probably within the last 20 million years
since geological evidence strongly indicates that the Pacific
salmon ancestors immigrated from the Atlantic (Behnke, 1990).

The American shad (*Alosa sapidissima*) shows a fascinating
continuum between semelparity and iteroparity: the more
southerly the latitude, the fewer are repeat spawners (Fig.
10.4) (Leggett & Carscaden, 1978). Other migratory fish also
show conditional semelparity (Finch, 1990, pp. 92–93).

In summary, these examples of marsupial mice and fish show
clearly that closely related organisms can have very different life
histories, in which the pacemakers for life span are
environmental.

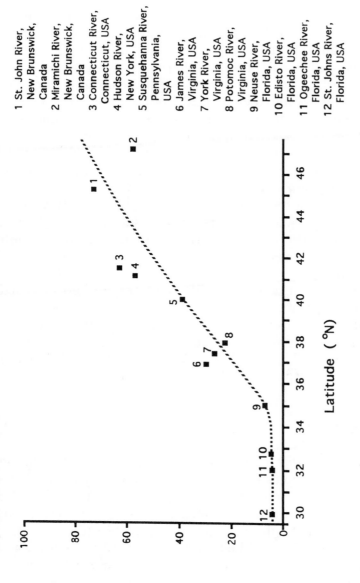

FIGURE 10.4 The American shad (*Alosa sapidissima*) shows a continuum between semelparity and iteroparity: the more southerly the latitude, the fewer are repeat spawners. Data of Leggett and Carscaden, 1978. (Redrawn from Finch, 1990, p. 93.)

Fruitflies

The fruitfly has recently shown us the ease with which genetic selection can change the reproductive schedule and the life span (Rose, 1991). In an important series of studies, Michael Rose and colleagues have sampled natural populations of the fruitfly *Drosophila melanogaster*. These flies were brought to the laboratory and then placed under artificial selection to breed lines of individuals that were still reproducing at ages when 95% of the group had died. Within 15 generations, the maximum life span of females was increased by 30% (Fig. 10.5). The success of these artificial selection experiments depended on the formation of new sets of alleles. Once life span was increased, it could be nonetheless reversed by selecting for flies with early reproduction. This reversal shows that the changes did not depend on new mutations, but rather on assembling new combinations of alleles from those that preexisted in the population.

The causes for changes in life span are not known. A likely possibility is some relationship to reproductive functions. For example, flies selected for greater life span and delayed senescence had smaller ovaries as adults and delayed peak egg production (Rose, 1984a,b,c; Luckinbill et al., 1984). These features of the reproductive schedule are under close hormonal control.

Honeybees

Honeybees (*Apis mellifica*) and many other social insects give wonderful examples of plasticity in life history in which individuals from the same batch of eggs may become either short-lived workers, with maximum life spans of months, or long-lived queens, with life spans of 5 or more years (Finch, 1990, pp. 67–72; Wilson, 1971; Winston, 1987) (Fig. 10.6). There is absolute certainty that both queens and workers have identical genomes. The choice is made by attending nurse bees, which feed the queen-destined larvae more often and with a special diet. Here we have an unequivocal example of selective gene

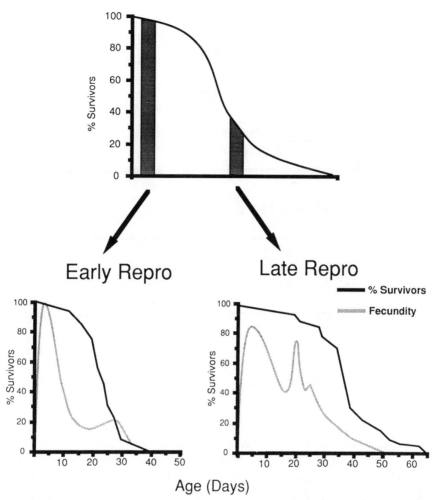

FIGURE 10.5 Michael Rose and colleagues have taken a sample from natural populations of the fruitfly *Drosophila melanogaster* and then selected for individuals that were still reproducing at ages when 95% of the group had died. Within 15 generations, the maximum life span of females was increased by 30%. (Redrawn from Rose et al., 1984.)

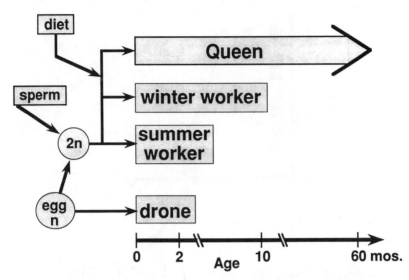

FIGURE 10.6 Honeybees (*Apic mellifica*), and many other social insects give wonderful examples of plasticity in life history, in which individuals from the same batch of eggs may become either short-lived workers with maximum life spans of months, or long-lived queens, with life spans of 5 or more years. (*Sources*: Finch, 1990, pp. 67–72; Wilson, 1971; Winston, 1987. Redrawn from Finch, 1990, p. 68.)

regulation during development that epigenetically sets the adult life span potential through anatomy and behavior. Not so incidently, queens provide another counter example to caloric restriction, since they require relatively large amounts of food to maintain their high daily production of eggs.

Worker honeybees show yet another type of plasticity in life history. Initially, workers remain in the hive, where they fly very little and mostly attend the feeding and grooming of the queen. However, at a certain age, which is influenced by population density, juvenile hormone levels raise in their hemolymph. This hormonal change stimulates workers to leave the hive and begin foraging flights (Fluri et al., 1982), a change to a far more dangerous occupation that is associated with accelerating mortality risks. Juvenile hormone, which is best known for its role in regulating development, has many roles and at this stage in the worker bee life history, functions as a death hormone, much as does cortisol in Pacific salmon.

EVOLUTIONARY THEORY PREDICTS A DIVERSITY IN PATTERNS OF AGING

Evolutionary theories of senescence generally emphasize how natural selection can be exerted on a gene pool despite the high rates of postmaturational mortality that characterize many species. The aggregate age-independent mortality rate may be so high from natural hazards irrespective of any senescence, such that only a small fraction can survive much beyond the first season of reproduction.

A major line of reasoning founded by Haldane (1941) considered that mouse strains with different hereditary diseases at mid-life are models for the escape of genotypes from natural selection if adverse effects are late in onset. Others subsequently argued that natural selection is weak against genotypes for chronic diseases and other dysfunctions that arise long after the start of reproduction (Medawar, 1952; Williams, 1957; Hamilton, 1966).

Quantitative arguments are based on the population models, such as the Euler-Lotka equation, in which the rate of population growth represents the balancing between mortality and fecundity. The extent of senescence according to this theory should be closely linked to adult phase mortality rates (Rose, 1991). These proposals lead to a major theoretical prediction that the high natural mortality rates of most populations allow the accumulation of genes in older age groups that cause age-correlated deteriorations or senescence, because so few survive to ages when these adverse genetic effects are manifested (Charlesworth, 1980, Rose, 1991). The outcome of this prediction is a major issue and conclusions are by no means straightforward or settled. Examples like the fulmar (Fig. 10.2) may be particulary challenging for despite high overall mortality rates, senescence has not been detected.

A corollary to the proposition that the force of selection diminishes with age, emphasized by Haldane, Medawar, Williams, and Rose is that genetically based manifestations of senescence should vary widely between species and within species. It is obvious that there are large variations between taxa in regard to developmental patterns, e.g., cell lineage determination, the onset of the zygote genomic functions, etc. Superimposed on species developmental differences may be even greater variations in senescence.

Evolutionary shifts in senescence and longevity are obvious in comparisons of the life histories, e.g., short-lived flies versus long-lived insect queens; mice versus elephants, etc. Population geneticists often view the evolution of senescence as part of the more general problem of genetic selection for life history. It is presumed that senescence is highly labile during evolution. Shortening or lengthening of life span, with acceleration or deceleration of senescence, may have occurred on innumerable occasions.

The examples of artificial selection for life span on the basis of reproductive schedule in *Drosophila* give strong support to this plasticity; the examples of short- and long-lived castes from the same genome in social insects show further that plasticity in life span can be a deeper trait in genetic coding that can operate epigenetically. It is unclear at this time to what either mechanism, genetic or epigenetic, accounts for the increase of human life expectancy during recent history.

HUMAN LIFE SPANS AND LIFE HISTORY PLASTICITY

Basis for Optimism

These examples from other animals suggest that there may be many aspects of human aging that are not inevitably programmed and that can be modified through epigenetic approaches. From many national populations, the mortality rate curves, when plotted semi-logarithmically show a quite consistent parallel shift to the right. For example, Figure 10.7 shows the mortality rates at very advanced ages in England and Wales, regraphed from Thatcher (1992). These other sources show, contrary to predictions by Fries (1980), that there is no hint of accelerating mortality at later ages such as would be required if the maximum human life span were fixed. While such data can not be extrapolated into the future, the demographics of life spans shows considerable plasticity, whether from genetic or epigenetic causes, just as observed in the examples given above. We may anticipate even further perturbations of mortality patterns at later ages, given a range of life-style and pharmacologic interventions that are practiced with ever increasing popularity.

A major set of phenomena is associated with the loss of estrogens during menopause. Consequences include acceleration of osteoporosis which is an important cause of spontaneous fractures in elderly women, atrophy of mucosa in the reproductive tract, hot flashes and increases of cardiovascular disease. This syndrome of estrogen deficits can be greatly modified by replacement of estrogens. Moreover, estrogen replacements reduce mortality from cardiovascular disease (reviewed in Henderson et al., 1993). Furthermore, combination oral contraceptives (COC) with a regimen of estrogens and progesterone considerably reduce the subsequent and age-related increase of cancer in breast, uterus, and ovaries (Henderson et al., 1993). Chemoprevention of these diverse age-related diseases in women doubtless involves several mechanisms. In reproductive tract cancers, the key to chemoprevention appears to be reduction of proliferation in hormone target tissues, whereas in the vascular system, hormonal chemoprevention may work by modifying the amounts of low and high density blood lipoproteins.

It is plausible that some combinations of steroids or steroid antagonists will be effective both in contraception and in reducing the risk of fractures, reproductive tract cancers, and vascular disease in women. Antiandrogens are already used as a chemopreventive for prostatic hypertrophy and cancer,

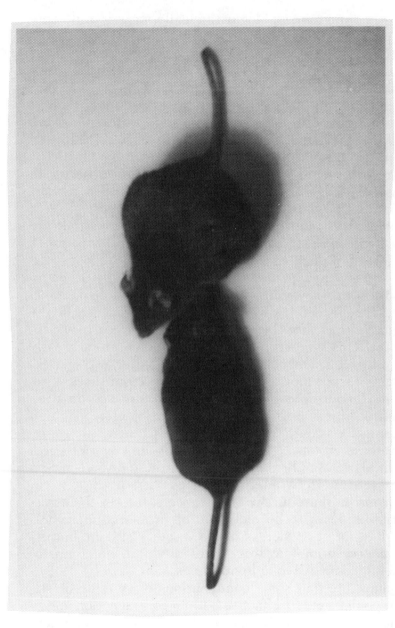

FIGURE 9.2 Two compound transgenic mice aged about 120 days. The mouse on the left received GCV, while the animal on the right received saline. Note the marked abdominal swelling in the placebo-treated mouse, indicative of advanced liver cancer.

e.g., Finasteride. These actions are epigenetic, since the target tissue responses depend on the selective regulation of gene activity.

Alzheimer's disease may also be viewed epigenetically, even in the familial autosomal dominant form. This perspective arises from considering Down's syndrome, which is caused by trisomy 21. Besides the developmental abnormalities that impair intelligence, virtually all Down's develop the neuropathology of Alzheimer's disease, with vascular amyloid, neuritic plaques, and cytokeletal abnormalities (Wisniewski et al., 1978; Mann, 1988). The cause of Alzheimer neuropathology in Down's is the imbalance of gene dose. Once we know which genes are crucial for the development of Alzheimer changes during Down's, it may be possible to intervene at the level of gene regulation in Alzheimer's disease.

As a last example, it is clear that diet can strongly influence health and other outcomes of aging at later ages (Weindruch & Walford, 1988). Diet is suspected in the lower incidence of breast cancer in Japan than in Japanese women in Los Angeles, who have the same incidence as local Caucasian (Henderson et al., 1984). Appropriate diets are well known to slow the course of hereditary type II diabetes and in common blood lipid disorders. Finally, caloric restriction slows the loss of ovarian oocytes in rodents (Nelson et al., 1985). Thus, even the fundamental ovarian clock of aging can be influenced by environmental means. These examples are selected from a major literature of experimental interventions that modify details of aging changes and, in the examples of diet restriction, also slow the mortality acceleration rate (Finch, 1990, pp. 506–510).

Basis for Caution

While there is no doubt that mammalian physiology allows great plasticity throughout development and into adult life, there are also damaging biochemical processes that have cumulative effects on many slowly replaced or unreplaceable

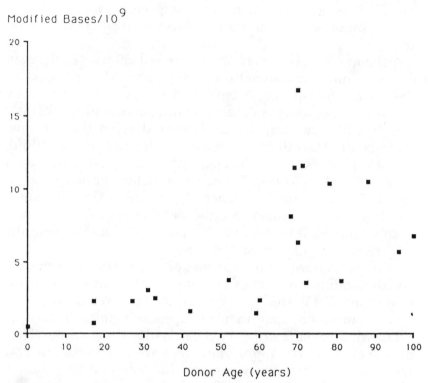

FIGURE 10.8   DNA adducts (covalently modified bases) in samples from the brains of neurologically normal individuals from Sweden. (*Source*: Randerath et al., 1992.)

molecules. DNA in many tissues is now recognized to accumulate covalent adducts, as shown in human brain DNA, where samples from older adults typically have about 10 modified bases per cell nucleus, or about 1 per 10,000 genes (Fig. 10.8) (Randerath et al., 1992). In some tissues with active cell proliferation, certain of these adducts are associated with chemical carcinogens (Liehr et al., 1986).

Mitochondrial DNA (mtDNA) deletions, however, imply a more general hazard to functions. Studies from several labs indicate progressive increases in mtDNA deletions (Pikó et al., 1988; Soong et al., 1992): dopaminergic rich regions of the human brain show the most marked increase at later ages, up to two hundredfold more than the cortex and cerebellum. About 5% of mitochondria may become damaged in the human basal ganglia during aging. Linnane et al. (1989) proposed that mtDNA damage causes significant deficits in oxidative phosphorylation with age. The association with dopamine suggests a link to oxidative damage, because dopamine metabolism produces free radicals. This regional vulnerability may also point the way to a neuropharmacology of mtDNA deletions. Long-term treatment with dopamine agonists which reduce synaptic dopamine protected the rat striatum against many aging changes; so far mtDNA has not been examined in these studies (Felton et al., 1992).

Oxidative damage to proteins is another slow outcome of aging and is clearly shown for proteins throughout the body (Finch, 1990, pp. 400–405; Stadtman, 1988; Smith et al., 1991). Glycation is one class of oxidative damage to proteins and occurs nonenzymatically from the chemical reaction of endogenous glucose with reactive groups on proteins. The products are often referred to as AGE, for advanced glycation endproducts (Lee & Cerami, 1988; Monnier et al., 1990). Diabetes with elevated blood glucose increases the extent of glycation (Schnider & Kohn, 1980; Lee & Cerami, 1988). Nonetheless, it should be possible to devise interventions for slowing the rate of glycation: birds have very high levels of blood glucose, which combined with their higher body temperatures, would predict extensive glycation (Monnier et al., 1990). No information is available on the extent of glycation in avian proteins.

CONCLUSIONS

Together, these examples are consistent with evolutionary views of the life span that require great temporal plasticity for selection on the basis of the reproductive schedule. The ultimate basis for all of these variations in life history is the maintenance of genomic totipotency, or the diploid genome inherited from parents and found in nearly all somatic cells. Apart from the erythrocytes, which lack a nucleus completely, or the B and T cells, which have rearranged genes for the immunoglobulins and the T-cell receptor, age changes in virtually all other cells should be modifiable or reversible by reprogramming the patterns of gene expression. Thus, we might calibrate the long-range goals for intervention by examining the tissues that show least age-related damage in the population that on the average maintains health to the greatest age. While there may be no total escape from the adverse experiences of aging at molecular and cellular levels, the extent of age-related change should in principal be as accessible to human intentions as is the range of different life histories in other animals that resulted from natural selection.

REFERENCES

Behnke, R.J. (1989): We're putting them back alive. *Trout* (Autumn).

Behnke, R.J. (1990): Interpreting the phylogeny of. Salvelinus. *Physiol.Ecol.Jpn., special issue, 1.*

Behnke, R.J. (1990): Still a rainbow by any other name. Why are rainbow trout now Oncorhynchus mykiss? Does this make them salmon? *Trout,42–45.*

Campbell, R.N. (1979): Ferox trout, Salmo trutta L., and charr, Salvelinus alpinus (L.), in Scottish lochs. *J.Fish.Biol.* 14: 1–29.

Comfort, A. (1979): *The Biology of Senescence*, 3rd ed. London: Churchill Livingston.

Diamond, J.M. (1982): Big-bang reproduction and aging in male marsupial mice. *Nature* 298: 115–116.

Fagerlund, U.H.M. (1967): Plasma cortisol concentration in relation to stress in adult sockeye salmon during the freshwater state of their life cycle. *Gen.Comp.Endocrinol.* 8: 197–207.

Farrer, L.A, Myers, R.H, Cupples, L.A, et al. (1990): Transmission and age at onset patterns in familial Alzheimer's disease: Evidence for heterogeneity. *Neurology* 40: 395–403.

Ferguson, A and Mason, F.M. (1981): Allozyme evidence for reproductively isolated sympatric populations of brown trout Salmo trutta L. in Lough Melvin, Ireland. *J.Fish.Biol.* 18: 629–642.

Finch, C.E. (1990): *Longevity, Senescence, and the Genome*, Chicago IL: University of Chicago Press.

Fluri, P, Luscher, M, Wille, H and Gerig, L. (1982): Changes in weight of the pharyngeal gland and haemolymph titres of juvenile hormone, protein, and vitellogenin in worker honey bees. *J.Insect Physiol.* 28: 61–68.

Fries, J.F. (1980): Aging, natural death, and the compression of morbidity. *N.Engl.J.Med.* 303: 130–135.

Gosden, R.G. (1985): *The Biology of Menopause: the Causes and Consequences of Ovarian Aging.* New York: Academic Press.

Haldane, J.B.S. (1942): *New Paths in Genetics*, London:Allen and Unwin.

Hamilton, K.E, Ferguson, A, Taggart, J.B, Tomasson, T, Walker, A and Fahy, E. (1989): Post-glacial colonization of brown trout, Salmo trutta L.: Ldh-5 as a phylogeographic marker locus. *J.Fish.Biol.* 35: 651–664.

Hamilton, W.D. (1966): The moulding of senescence by natural selection. *J.Theoret.Biol.* 12: 12–45.

Henderson, B.E., Pike, M.C., and Ross, R.K. (1984): Epidemiology and risk factors. In, *Breast cancer: Diagnosis and Management.*, G. Bonadonna (Ed.), pp. 15–33, New York: Wiley and Sons.

Henderson, B.E., Ross, R.K., and Pike, M.C. (1993): Hormonal chemoprevention of cancer in women. *Science* 259: 633–638.

Kanisto, V. (1988) On the survival of centenarians and the span of life. *Pop. Studies* 42: 389–406.

Lee, A.K. and Cockburn, A. (1985) *Evolutionary Ecology of Marsupials*, New York:Cambridge Univ. Press.

Lee, A.T. and Cerami, A. (1990): Modifications of proteins and nucleic acids by reducing sugars. In *Handbook of the Biology of Aging*, 3rd ed., E.L. Schneider and J.W. Rowe (eds.), pp. 116–130, San Diego: Academic Press.

Leggett, W.C and Carscadden, J.E. (1978): Latitudinal variation in reproduction characteristics of American shad (Alosa sapidissima): Evidence for population-specific life history strategies in fish. *J.Fish.Res.Bd.Can.* 35: 1469–1478.

Liehr, J.G, Avitts, T.A, Randerath, E and Randerath, K. (1986): Estrogen-induced endogenous DNA adduction: Possible mechanism of hormonal cancer. *Proc.Natl.Acad.Sci.* 83: 5301–5305.

Linnane, A.W, Marzuki, S, Ozawa, T and Tanaka, M. (1989): Mitochondrial DNA mutations as an important contributor to age-ing and degenerative diseases. *Lancet* 1: 642–645.

Luckinbill, L.S, Arking, R, Clare, M.J, Cirocco, W.C and Buck, S.A. (1984): Selection for delayed senescence in Drosophila melano-gaster. *Evolution* 38: 996–1003.

Mann, D.M.A. (1988): The pathological association between Down syndrome and Alzheimer disease. *Mech.Age.Dev.* 43: 99–136.

Medawar, P.B. (1952) *An Unsolved Problem of Biology*, London:H.K.Lewis.

Monnier, V.M, Sell, D.R, Miyata, S and Nagara, R.H. The Maillard re-action as a basis for a theory of aging. In: *Proceedings of the 4th International Symposium on the Maillard Reaction, P. A. Finot (ed.)*, Basel: Birkhausert-Verlag, 1990, p. 393–414. Adv.

Nelson, J.F. and Felicio, L.S. (1985): Reproductive aging in the female: An etiological perspective. *Rev.Biol.Res.Aging* 2: 251–314.

Ollason, J.C. and Dunnet, G.M. Variation in breeding success in fulmars. (1988) In: *Reproductive Success. Studies of Individual Variation in Contrasting Breeding Systems, T. H. Clutton-Brock (ed.)*, Chicago: Univ. of Chicago Press, p. 263–278.

Pikó, L., Hougham, A.J., and Bulpitt, K.J. (1988): Studies of sequence heterogeneity of mitochondrial DNA in mouse and rat : evi-dence for an increased frequency of deletions/additions with aging. *Mech. Aging. Devel.* 43: 279–293.

Randerath, K., Putnam, K.L., Osterburg, H.H., Johnson, S.A., Mor-gan, D.G., and Finch, C.E. (1992): Age-dependent increases of DNA adducts (I-compounds) in human and rat brain DNA. *Mu-tation Res.* 295: 11–18.

Robertson, O.H, Krupp, M.A, Thomas, S.F, Favour, C.B, Hane, S and Wexler, B.C. (1961): Hypoadrenocorticism in spawning migra-tory and non-migratory rainbow trout: Salmo gairdnerii. *Gen-.Comp.Endocrinol.* 1: 473–484.

Robertson, O.H, Wexler, B.C and Miller, B.F. (1961): Degenerative changes in the cardiovascular system of the spawning Pacific salmon (Oncorhynchus tshawytscha). *Circ.Res.* 9: 826–834.

Robertson, O.H. (1957): Survival of precociously mature king salmon (Oncoryhynchus tshawytscha) after spawning. *Calif. Fish and Game* 43: 119–130.

Robertson, O.H. (1961): Prolongation of the lifespan of kokanee salmon (O. nerka kennerlyi) by castration before beginning de-velopment. *Proc.Natl.Acad.Sci.* 47: 609–621.

Rose, M.R, Dorey, M.L, Coyle, A.M and Service, P.M. (1984): The morphology of postponed senescence in Drosophila melanogaster. *Can.J.Zool.* 62: 1576–1580.

Rose, M.R. (1984a): Laboratory evolution of postponed senescence in Drosophila melanogaster. *Evolution* 38: 1004–1010.

Rose, M.R. (1984b): The evolution of animal senescence. *Can.J.Zool.* 62: 1661–1667.

Rose, M.R. (1984c): Genetic covariation in Drosophila life history: Untangling the data. *Am.Nat.* 123: 565–569.

Rose, M.R. *The Evolutionary Biology of Aging*, Oxford:Oxford Univ. Press, 1991.

Rose, M.R., Dorey, M.L., Coyle, A.M. and Service, P.M. (1984): The morphology of postponed senescence in Drosophila melano-gaster. *Can.J.Zool.* 62: 1576–1580.

Saunders, R.L and Farrell, A.P. (1988): Coronary arteriosclerosis in Atlantic salmon. *Arteriosclerosis* 8: 378–384.

Simms, H.S. (1945) Logarithmic increase of mortality as a manifes-tation of aging. *J. Gerontol.* 1: 13–25.

Smith, C.D., Carney, J.M., Satrke-Reed, P.E., Oliver, C.N., Stadtman, E.R., Floyd, R.A., and Markesbery, W.R. (1991): Excess brain protein oxidation and enzyme dysfunction in normal aging and in Alzheimer disease. *PNAS* 88: 10540–01543.

Soong, N.W., Hinton, D.R., Cortopassi, G. and Arnheim, N. (1992): Mosaicism for a specific somatic mitochondrial DNA mutation in adult human brain. *Nature Genetics* 2: 318–323.

Stadtman, E.R. (1988): Minireview: Protein modification in aging. *J. Gerontol.* 43: B112-B120.

Thatcher, A.R. (1992): Trends in numbers and mortality at high ages in England and Wales. *Pop. Studies* 46: 411–426.

Van Dyke, J. and Fobes, N. (1993): Long journey of the Pacific salmon. *Nat.Geographic* July: 3–37.

van Overbeeke, A.P. and McBride, J.R. (1971):Histological effects of 11-ketotestosterone, 17a-methyltestosterone, estradiol cyprio-nate, and cortisol on the interrenal tissues, thyroid gland, and pituitary gland of the gonadectomized sockeye salmon (Oncor-hynchus nerka). *J. Fish. Res. Bd. Can.* 28: 477–484.

Weindruch, R.H. and Walford, R.L. (1988): *The Retardation of Aging and Disease by Dietary Restriction.* Springfield IL: C.C. Thomas.

Williams, G.C. (1957): Pleiotropy, natural selection, and the evolu-tion of senescence. *Evolution* 11: 398–411.

Wilson, E.O. *The Insect Societies*, Cambridge, MA:Belknap Press, 1971.

Winston, M.L. *The Biology of the Honey Bee*, Cambridge, MA:Harvard Univ. Press, 1987.

Wisniewski, K, Howe, J, Williams, D.G and Wisniewski, H.M. (1978): Precocious aging and dementia in patients with Down's syndrome. *Biol.Psychiatry* 13: 619–31.

Brain and Life Span in Catarrhine Primates

11

John Allman

INTRODUCTION

In haplorhine primates (tarsiers, new world monkeys, old world monkeys, apes and humans) there is a strong positive correlation between brain weight and life span when the effect of body size is removed (Allman, McLaughlin, & Hakeem, 1993a). This correlation has been observed for both maximum recorded lifespan for each species and for average age of first reproduction in females for each species. The volumes of many brain structures are also strongly correlated with lifespan when the effect of body size is removed (Allman, McLaughlin, & Hakeem, 1993b). In this paper I explore the linkage between specific brain structures and longevity in our close relatives, the catarrhine primates (old world monkeys, apes, humans). The catarrhine brain structures that are highly correlated with life span, such as the cerebellum, amygdala, hypothalamus and neocortex, may be particularly important in sustaining survival and thus are relevant to the formulation of strategies for delaying dysfunction in later life in humans.

METHODS

I used the maximum recorded life span because it should measure, under ideal circumstances, the genetic potential for longevity for each species. Comparable data for a large number of species are not available for average life span. My colleagues and I collected a database of life spans for catarrhine primate species by zoos and research institutions throughout the world (Hakeem et al., 1994). Our queries were guided by records from the International Species Inventory System (ISIS) and by the records of Marvin Jones, Registrar of the San Diego Zoological Society. Many of the long-lived animals were born in the wild, and their age at acquisition could only be estimated. We accepted the zoos' estimates of the ages at which they were acquired for immature animals. For animals acquired from the wild as adults, we used as the value for adult age, the average age of females at first reproduction from a table by Ross (1988). The maximum documented human life span is 120.6 years (MacFarland, 1992); however, this is based on a population about a million times larger than for any non-human primate. Therefore I used a value for a contemporary human population more nearly comparable in size to the populations of non-human primates sampled. In a sample of 1000 obituary notices recently published from August 1991 through June 1993 in the *Los Angeles Times* , the longest lived individual was 105 years old (anonymous, 1992).

Using brain and body weights obtained from a database compiled by Prof. Bob Martin, we tested the hypothesis that brain weight is correlated with life span when the effect of body weight is removed. We also used data from Stephan and his collaborators (Baron et al., 1983; Frahm et al., 1982, 1984; Matano et al., 1985 ; Stephan et al., 1981, 1982, 1984, 1987) on body weights and the volumes of various brain structures to determine which structures are correlated with life span. Since life span is correlated with body weight (Allman, McLaughlin, & Hakeem, 1993a), it was necessary to remove the effect of body weight to observe the net effect of variation in the size of the brain and its components. To remove the effect of body weight by the *residuals* methods, we plotted the base 10 logarithm of the parameter in question (brain weight or life-span, for example) against the base 10 logarithm of the body weight. The distance in the y dimension between the least-squares regression line and each data point was added to 1, giving a value > 1 for points the fall above the line and < 1 for points that fall below the line. This gives the *residual* value of this parameter for each species. In other words, I sought to determine whether a species that lived longer than one would expect for its body weight had brain or brain structure that was commensurately larger than would be expected for its body weight. I also used the method of partial correlations to remove the effect of body size on the log transformed data. In virtually every case the partial correlation was equal or higher than the residual correlation. The data was analyzed with the assistance of the computer programs Systat and Statview.

RESULTS

In previous work we found that the brain weight residuals and life span residuals were correlated in haplorhine primates (tarsiers, new world monkeys, old world monkeys, apes and humans) ($N = 49$, $r = 0.657$, $p = 0.001$), but not in strepsirhine primates (lorises and lemurs) ($N = 16$, $r = 0.005$, $p = 0.838$) (Allman et al., 1993a). Table 11.1 contains the correlations for the brain and many of its components for catarrhine primates. The most strongly correlated structure is the cerebellum (see also Fig. 11.1). The second, third and fourth structures are different layers of neocortex for which the sample size (5 species) was too small to achieve statistical significance. The next most strongly correlated structures is the hypothalamus (see also Fig. 11.2). The next six structures are all telencephalic, which generally are well-correlated except for the hippocampus and peripheral olfactory structures. In general, sensory structures such as the eye surface, lateral geniculate nucleus, primary visual cortex, vestibular nuclei, ol-

TABLE 11.1 Correlations Between Brain Structure (and other measures) Residuals and Life Span Residuals in Catarrhine Primates (Correlations with *p* Values of Less Than 0.05 are Printed in Boldface)

Structure	number of species	r	p
Cerebellum, whole	**14**	**0.873**	**<0.001**
Neocortex, lamina 1	5	0.838	0.082
Neocortex, gray matter	5	0.827	0.090
Neocortex, laminae 2-6	5	0.825	0.091
Hypothalamus	**8**	**0.824**	**0.012**
Prepiriform cortex	**13**	**0.769**	**0.00**
Septum	**13**	**0.756**	**0.003**
Piriform Lobe	**13**	**0.744**	**0.004**
Olfactory Tubercle	**13**	**0.741**	**0.004**
Amygdala, corticobasolateral complex	**13**	**0.738**	**0.004**
Amgdala, whole	**12**	**0.726**	**0.008**
Whole brain, Stephan brain weight	**14**	**0.722**	**0.004**
Thalamus	**8**	**0.718**	**0.046**
Neocortex, white matter	5	0.7	0.182
Subcommissural body	**9**	**−0.690**	**0.040**
Telencephalon	**14**	**0.661**	**0.010**
Amgdala, centromedial complex	**13**	**0.656**	**0.015**
Triangular nucleus of the septum	9	−0.651	0.058
Female age at first reproduction	**30**	**0.637**	**<0.001**
Subthalamus	8	0.637	0.091
Globus pallidus	8	0.635	0.092
Neocortex, including white matter	**14**	**0.630**	**0.016**
Ventral pons	**13**	**0.629**	**0.021**
Substantia innominata	**13**	**0.617**	**0.025**
Mesencephalon	**14**	**0.613**	**0.020**
Trigeminal complex	**13**	**0.592**	**0.033**
Striatum	**14**	**0.573**	**0.032**
Cerebellar nuclei, lateral	**13**	**0.573**	**0.041**
Retrobulbar cortex	**13**	**0.560**	**0.047**
Diencephalon	14	0.531	0.051
Amygdala, magnocellular part of basal nucleus	13	0.52	0.067
Primary visual cortex gray matter, laminae 2-6	5	−0.4467	0.432
Vestibular complex, superior nucleus	13	0.349	0.243
Subfornical body	9	−0.345	0.363
Medial habenular nucleus	9	−0.341	0.370
Vestibular complex, lateral nucleus	13	−0.307	0.308
Hippocampus	14	0.295	0.306
Lateral olfactory tract	13	0.260	0.391
Cerebellar nuclei, total	13	0.258	0.395

(continued)

TABLE 11.1 (*Continued*)

Structure	number of species	r	p
Basal metabolic rate	7	−0.253	0.585
Cerebellar nuclei, interpositus	13	−0.240	0.430
Cerebellar nuclei, medial	13	−0.194	0.526
Olfactory bulb, main	13	0.166	0.588
Vestibular complex, inferior nucleus	13	−0.141	0.646
Anterior commissure	13	0.137	0.655
Primary visual cortex gray matter	10	−0.135	0.710
Primary visual cortex, total	10	−0.11	0.753
Medulla	14	0.114	0.698
Pineal	9	0.111	0.776
Eye surface, half	19	−0.109	0.658
Primary visual cortex gray matter, lamina 1	5	−0.105	0.868
Primary visual cortex, white matter	10	−0.079	0.829
Testes weight	19	0.066	0.789
Lateral geniculate nucleus	11	−0.054	0.874
Vestibular complex, total	13	−0.050	0.872
Vestibular complex, medial nucleus	13	−0.006	0.985

factory bulb, and lateral olfactory tract are not significantly correlated. However, in striking exception to the other sensory structures, higher olfactory structures such as the olfactory tubercule, piriform lobe and prepiriform cortex are well correlated (see Fig. 11.3). One structure, the subcommissural body, is significantly *negatively* correlated with life span. Many more individual brain structures are correlated with life span in catarrhine primates (old world monkeys, apes and humans) than in other primate groups. There are 20 correlated structures in catarrhines, whereas there are only 5 in platyrhines (new world monkeys) and 3 in strepsirhines (lorises and lemurs). The number of species sampled in the 3 groups was about the same and thus variations in sample size do not appear to account for this difference. Thus the brain correlations with life span tend to be stronger in our close relatives. The correlation between whole brain weight and life span is extremely strong for our own species and our closest relatives, gorillas, orangutans, chimpanzees ($N = 4$, $r = .997$,

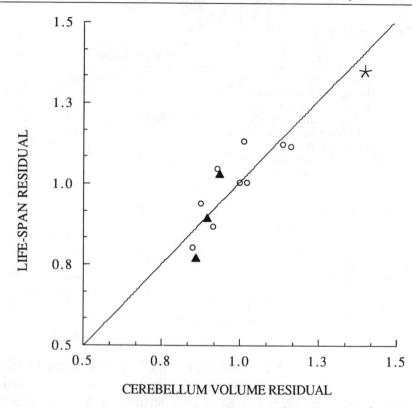

FIGURE 11.1 The relationship between cerebellar volume and lifespan in catarrhine primates with the effect of body size removed (see Methods section). The number of species plotted is 14; $r=0.873$; $p=<0.001$. The slope of the major axis regression is 2.314. The solid triangles indicate leave-eating species; the circles indicate fruit-eating species; the star is *Homo sapiens*.

$p = 0.006$). The same appears to be true for separate brain structures in these primates. Although data are available for only 8 structures, 7 are significantly correlated with life span (see Table 11.2). The only exception is the hippocampus which is almost significant ($p = 0.07$).

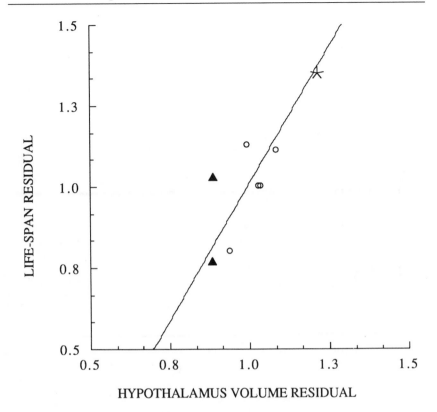

FIGURE 11.2 The relationship between hypothalamic volume and lifespan with the effect of body size removed in catarrhine primates (see Methods section). The number of species plotted is 8; $r=0.824$; $p=0.012$. The slope of the major axis regression is 3.778. The solid triangles indicate leaf-eating species; the circles indicate fruit-eating species; the triangle is *Homo sapiens*.

DISCUSSION

Longevity in the Wild

We have very little information on the longevity of primates in the wild because this would require sustained observations

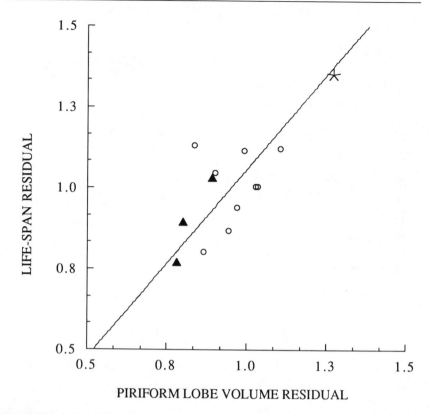

FIGURE 11.3 The relationship between piriform lobe volume and lifespan with the effect of body size removed (see Methods section). The number of species plotted is 13; $r=0.7741$; $p=0.004$. The slope of the major axis regression is 2.635. The solid triangles indicate leaf-eating species; the circles indicate fruit-eating species; the triangle is *Homo sapiens*.

of wild populations for many decades. My data are based on captive primates; however the few very long-term studies of primates living under natural conditions indicate that some individuals live into extreme old age in the wild. One might think that primates living in zoos would have longer maximum life spans than those living in the wild, but long-term observational data suggest that the maximum life spans for zoo-living and wild primates may be about the same. Glander (personal communication) has measured tooth wear in a wild population of 580 howler monkeys (*Alouatta palliata*) in Costa Rica since 1970. Twelve of these monkeys have been under continuous observation since 1970. In these old monkeys, which he estimates to be between 24 and 28 years old, the teeth are all worn down to the gum line. The maximum life spans recorded for captive *Aoulatta* species range from 20 to 28 years and thus appear to be fairly close to the longevity in the wild (Hakeem et al., 1994).

Goodall (1986) observed 11 chimpanzees at Gombe from 1965 through 1983 that she considered old. One of these was Flo, who was a very successful individual with high-ranking offspring, Figan and Fifi (see Fig. 11.4). Flo's teeth were worn down to the gum line and Goodall estimated her age 4 years before her death as "certainly more than 40." Her status and aggressive personality were strong factors in Figan and Fifi's achievement of high rank. Flo remained reproductive into old age, but her last 2 offspring Flint and Flame did not flourish. The infant Flame died during her mother's illness. Flint, though more than 8 years old at the time of his mother's death, was unable to survive without her support.

Thus the limited data available from primates living in natural conditions indicate that some individuals live into robust old age. These observations suggest that the parent's healthy longevity contributes to the reproductive success of their offspring, and is likely to be a factor in the evolution of life-span sustaining mechanisms in higher primates. The parent's longevity may be particularly important in catarrhine primates, and especially in apes and humans, because development is slow, the period of dependence on the parents is long, and even in adulthood social status of the offspring may be closely linked to maternal status. These factors may be linked to the nearly perfect correlations between brain and most brain structures and lifespan in the group comprised of gorillas, orangutans, chimpanzees and humans (see Table 11.2).

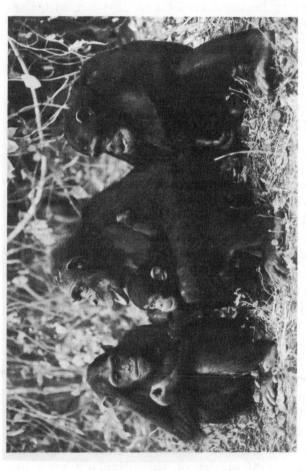

FIGURE 11.4 Flo, a successful elderly chimpanzee, and her family. From left to right: Fifi, Flint, Flo, and Figan. Goodall (1986) estimated Flo to be "certainly more than 40 years old"; her teeth were worn down to the gum line more than 8 years before her death. On the basis of her skeletal remains, Zihlman et al. (1990) estimated that she lived to the age of 43. Her offspring, Fifi and Figan achieved high status. Although Flint was 8 at the time of Flo's death; he was still very dependent on her and was unable to survive without her. (Reprinted by permission of the publishers from THE CHIMPANZEES OF GOMBE by Jane Goodall, Cambridge, Mass.: Harvard University Press, copyright © 1986 by the President and Fellows of Harvard College.)

TABLE 11.2 Correlations Between Brain Structure Residuals and Life Span Residuals From Gorillas, Chimpanzees, Orangutans and Humans (Correlations with _p_ Values of Less Than 0.05 are Printed in Boldface.)

Brain Structure	r	p
brain (whole)	**0.997**	**0.006**
striatum	**0.994**	**0.010**
mesencephalon	**0.993**	**0.012**
diencephalon	**0.989**	**0.016**
neocortex, incl. white matter	**0.988**	**0.017**
telencephalon	**0.988**	**0.018**
medulla	**0.987**	**0.019**
hippocampus	0.942	0.070

Cerebellum and Life Span

The volume of the cerebellum is very well correlated with life span ($r = .873$) (see Fig. 11.1). The size of the cerebellum alone can account for 76% of the variance in life span of catarrhine species when the effect of body size is removed. There are many studies which indicate that the cerebellum is particularly vulnerable to the deleterious effects of aging. For example, in studies of large populations of humans, there is an approximately 20% average loss in the volume of the cerebellum between young adulthood and very old age (Hall et al., 1975) versus only a 10% loss in the volume of the whole brain (Dekaban & Sadowsky, 1978). The cerebellar cortex is packed with small granule cells that comprise about half the neurons in the brain. A morphologically distinct population of very large neurons arranged in an almost crystalline array, the Purkinje cells, are the sole line of communication to the rest of the brain from the huge population of cells in the cerebellar cortex.

There are many studies in a variety of mammals, going back as far as 1894, indicating the loss of Purkinje cells with advancing age (Ellis, 1920a,b; Hall et al., 1975; Rogers et al., 1984; Torvik & Torp, 1986; Torvik et al., 1986; Sturrock, 1989). Purkinje cells also are especially vulnerable to a variety of physiologically abnormal conditions such as chronic alcohol intoxication (Torvik et al., 1982), jaundice (Takagishi & Yamamura, 1989), anoxia (Brierley & Graham, 1984), and cancer in non-brain organs (Torvik et al., 1986). These effects are exacerbated with increasing age (Torvik et al., 1986). Purkinje cells have extensive dendritic arborizations, and the fine tertiary dendrites, which receive the synaptic contacts from the multitude of granule cell axons, appear to be particularly vulnerable in aging (Rogers et al., 1984; Quackenbush et al., 1990). As might be expected from the dying back of the Purkinje dendrites, there is age-related loss of granule-Purkinje cell synapses (Zornetzer et al., 1981; Glick & Bondareff, 1979). Physiological studies also reveal that the strength of the connectivity between the granule cells and the Purkinje cells declines with age (Rogers et al., 1981). Purkinje cells fire continuously at a high rate, however firing rate tends to become more irregular with age (Rogers, 1988). The high firing rate is probably related to the fact that the Purkinje cell influence on other neurons is entirely inhibitory; thus to communicate effectively they must be continuously active. This continuous high level of activity may make the Purkinje cells particularly vulnerable to a wide variety of physiologically abnormal states. In primates living in their natural habitats, these abnormal states might be induced by disease or by the dietary ingestion of plant toxins during the course of life. The computational architecture of the cerebellar cortex with its sole output, the Purkinje cells being solely inhibitory, creates a bottleneck that is especially vulnerable in aging.

Purkinje cell density in rabbits is closely correlated ($r = .79$) with the rate of acquisition of the auditory conditioned eyeblink response, a model for classical conditioning (Woodruff-Pak et al., 1990). In both rabbits and human subjects, the eyeblink response declines with age (Woodruff-Pak et al., 1988; Woodruff-Pak & Thompson, 1988), which suggests that this particular form of motor learning is related to integrity of the Purkinje cell population and declines with the loss of this population.

In addition to the loss of Purkinje cells, parts of the cerebellum undergo substantial age-related reduction in size. Data from a recent magnetic resonance imaging study indicate that there is a 25% to 30% reduction in the cross sectional area of the declive, folium, tuber and pyramis lobes of the cerebellar vermis measured in the midsagittal plane from ages 20 to 80 years (Raz et al., 1992). The more ventral segments of the vermis, the lingula-centralis and uvula-nodulus, showed no significant age-related loss in cross-sectional area. Degeneration was also reported to be more severe in the dorsal vermis in histological studies (Torvik et al., 1986). Thus the more phylogenetically recent parts of the cerebellar vermis, which mature later and receive more extensive neocortical connections, are the most vulnerable to the effects of aging (Raz et al., 1992).

I speculate that in the course of life, catarrhine primates are likely to ingest toxins or suffer pathophysiological states that would result in the loss of Purkinje cells and cerebellar mass. The consequent loss of sensory-motor coordination would be strongly selected against in these mainly tree dwelling primates. Thus the size of the cerebellum may be genetically linked to other factors governing life span so as to compensate for a certain level of probable exposure to damage during the course of life. In other words, it would be pointless to have an animal that in all other respects was capable of long survival, but fell from the trees at an early age because of cerebellar dysfunction.

The computational architecture of the cerebellum creates a linkage that is highly susceptible to dysfunction in the aging process. Because the Purkinje cells are the sole output of the cerebellar cortex and because this output is entirely inhibitory, the Purkinje cells must maintain a high level of activity and are especially vulnerable. One of the most debilitating losses of function in the elderly are the deficits of sensory-motor coordination that result in falls and fear of falling (Tideiksaar & Fletcher, 1989). Purkinje cell loss and cerebellar atrophy are likely to be a significant factors contributing to this loss of function. It is conceivable that strategies can be developed to prevent this loss in the elderly. We are fortunate that there are good animal models of age-related Purkinje cell loss that could be used to determine how to ameliorate this condition.

The Brain as a Homeostatic Buffer against Environmental Variation

The brain enhances survival by serving as a buffer against perturbations that would disrupt the homeostasis of the organism; these perturbations can be either internal or external to the organism (Sacher, 1975; Allman et al., 1993a). In a broad sense homeostasis between the animal and its environment and homeostasis within the organism both involve the continuous flow of energy and information crucial for survival.

With respect to the external environment, animals that have longer life spans are more likely during the course of their lives to suffer severe crises (such as shortages in normally used food resources) than are animals with shorter life spans (Allman, McLaughlin, & Hakeem, 1993a). For endotherms, there are essentially two ways to deal with food shortages resulting from environmental fluctuations. The first is to live off of energy stored in fat and down-regulate metabolism; the second is to store information about the environment and develop cognitive strategies so that the organism is able to switch to alternative food resources. All endotherms use both solutions to some extent, but many animals clearly specialize in one or the other. Hibernating animals (for example, bears and fat-tailed dwarf lemurs) represent the first solution while higher primates have relied more on the second solution.

There appears to be a link between the genetic mechanisms that control life span and the mechanisms controlling the growth of the brain such that there is more growth of specific structures in longer lived species (Allman, McLaughlin, & Hakeem, 1993a,b). The observed correlation in neocortical size represents the capacity to store information about the environment and develop cognitive strategies. Because of the magnitude of the neocortex in higher primates, the neocortical correlation is largely responsible for the correlation found for the entire brain in this group. The olfactory cortical structures are also well correlated with life span. These structures are probable sites for the formation and storage of olfactory memory (Haberly & Bower, 1989), and thus may be particularly important for the animal's knowledge of food resources. The cortical structures are the locus of the degenerative changes in Alzheimer's disease, which, because of its enormous clinical, social and economic importance, is the focus of major efforts to determine its cause and ameliorate its consequences.

The same argument holds for maintaining homeostasis in the internal milieu. Animals that have longer life spans are more likely to suffer severe crises than are animals with shorter life spans. The amygdala and hypothalamus are involved in maintaining physiological homeostasis. It is possible that the large size of these structures in the longer lived species may be due to more elaborate neural mechanisms for physiological homeostasis in these species. Alternatively, the larger size may represent reserve capacity of neurons so that the organism can sustain the loss of neurons over time without catastrophic loss of function, in manner analogous to the hypothesis previously advanced for the cerebellum.

The amygdala and hypothalamus may participate directly in the regulation of life span. For example, genetically programed age-specific cell death in the amygdala or hypothalamus could disrupt physiological homeostasis and cause the organism to self-destruct. This could be a late expression of selective neuron death that shapes the developing nervous system (Williams & Herrup, 1988). Although it by no means proves this hypothesis, it is intriguing that the main brain structure known to control temporal activity cycles, the suprachiasmatic nucleus of the hypothalamus, does exhibit substantial neuron death, which contrasts with the nearby supraoptic and paraventricular nuclei in which the adult neuron populations are maintained in the normal elderly and Alzheimer's patients (Swaab et al., 1993). The number of neurons in the suprachiasmatic nucleus is significantly reduced in individuals over 80 years of age as compared with younger subjects (Mirmiran et al., 1992). There is a significant further reduction in Alzheimer's patients as compared to the non-demented population over 80 years old (Goudsmit et al., 1992; Mirmiran et al., 1992).

The suprachiasmatic nucleus receives retinal input and regulates circadian and seasonal changes in physiological function (Moore, 1992; Hofman et al., 1993). There is a tendency for circadian rhythms to be disrupted in the elderly, and the effect is much stronger in Alzheimer's patients, who often have fragmented sleep patterns and nocturnal wandering (Mirmiran et al., 1992). Sleep-wakefulness rhythms improved and wandering was reduced in Alzheimer's patients following exposure to bright light for 2 hours each morning (Okawa et al., 1991). Thus there is a simple strategy for ameliorating this serious dysfunction in the elderly. Finally, since the suprachiasmatic nucleus is involved in the regulation of daily and seasonal activity cycles, it is possible that this or related hypothalamic structures may participate in the regulation of the whole life cycle.

The subcommissural body is significantly *negatively* correlated with life span. There is evidence for the participation of this structure in the regulation of salt-water homeostasis via interactions with the adrenals and in the cyclic release of gonadotrophin from the anterior pituitary (Sever et al., 1987; Limonta et al., 1982), both of which functions could be involved in the aging process.

SUMMARY

The brain and especially some of its components are linked to life span in higher primates when the statistical effect of body size is removed. The cerebellum, cerebral cortex and hypothalamus are especially well correlated; sensory structures tend not to be correlated. The relationship between brain and life span is particularly strong in our closest relatives, humans and the great apes where the correlation is nearly perfect ($r=0.997$). In humans and great apes, brain structures are also very strongly correlated with life span. In this group, seven of the eight brain structures for which data are available are significantly correlated. The especially strong correlations in humans and great apes may be due to the long period of parental dependence in these species and adapative value of having parental support even in adulthood in these species.

There are at least three general theories to explain why longer lived species have larger brains. The first is that the brain and its components serve to maintain homeostasis and thus enhance survival. The second is that the brain, or specific crucial brain components in long-lived species, has a reserve capacity of extra neurons that enhance survival to various forms of trauma and pathophysiological states. The third is that the brain and its components are subject to programmed cell death in adulthood and old age that is part of the whole ontogenetic cycle and that hypothalamic mechanisms may play a particularly important role in this cycle.

There are a number of ways in which these findings can contribute to delaying dysfunction in the elderly. There appear to be crucial neural populations, such as the Purkinje cells of the cerebellum, that are particularly vulnerable and strategies may be developed to prevent their loss or to enhance the functioning of the survivors. Hypothalamic mechanisms may be keys to the aging process and should receive greater investigation.

ACKNOWLEDGEMENTS

I thank the 138 zoos and research institutions who kindly provided primate life span data, and especially Mr. Marvin Jones, Registrar of the Zoological Society of San Diego, for his tireless help. I thank Prof. Bob Martin for kindly providing his unpublished data base of body and brain weights. I thank Ms. Atiya Hakeem, Ms. Gisela Sandoval, Mr. Todd McLaughlin, and Mr. Christopher Alexander for their valuable assistance in data collection and statistical analysis. Support for this research was provided by a grant from the Howard Hughes Medical Institute through the Undergraduate Biological Sciences Education Program and by grants from the National Institute on Aging, the McDonnell-Pew Program in Cognitive Neuroscience, and the Hixon Professorship.

REFERENCES

Allman, J., McLaughlin, T., and Hakeem, A. (1993a) Brain weight and life-span in primate species, *Proc. Natl. Acad. Sci.* 90: 118–122.

Allman, J., McLaughlin, T., and Hakeem, A. (1993b) Brain structures and life-span in primate species, *Proc. Natl. Acad. Sci.* 90: 3559–3563.

Anonymous (1992) Obituary for Annie Lloyd Welbourn, *Los Angeles Times*, May 31.

Baron, G., Frahm, H., Bhatnagar, K., Kunwar, P., and Stephan, H. (1983) Comparison of brain structure volumes in Insectivores and Primates. III. Main olfactory bulb (MOB), *J. Hirnforsch.* 24:551–568.

Brierley, J., and Graham, D. (1984) Hypoxia and vascular disorders of the central nervous system, In: Adams, J., Corsellis, J., and Duchen, L., (eds.) *Greenfield's Neuropathology*, John Wiley, New York, pp. 125–207.

Dekaban, A., Sadowsky, D. (1978) Changes in brain weight during the span of human life: relation of brain weights to body height and body weights, *Ann. Neurol.*, 4:343–356.

Ellis, R. (1920a) Norms for some structural changes in the human cerebellum from birth to old age, *J. Comp. Neurol.* 32:1–32.

Ellis, R. (1920b) A preliminary quantitative study of the Purkinje cells in normal, subnormal, and senescent human cerebella with some notes on functional localization, *J. Comp. Neurol.* 32: 229–252.

Frahm, H., Stephan, H., and Baron, G. (1984) Comparison of brain structure volumes in insectivores and primates. V. Area striata, *J. Hirnforsch.* 25:537–557.

Frahm, H., Stephan, H., and Stephan, M. (1982) Comparison of brain structure volumes in insectivores and primates. I. Neocortex, *J. Hirnforsch.* 23, 375–38.

Glick, R. and Bondareff, W. (1979) Loss of synapses in the cerebellar cortex of the rat, *J. Gereontol.* 34:818–822.

Goodall, Jane (1986) *The Chimpanzees of Gombe*, Harvard University Press, Cambridge.

Goudsmit, E., Neijmeijer-Leloux, Swaab, D. (1992) The human hypothalmo-neurohypophyseal system in relation to development, aging and Alzheimer's disease, *Prog. Brain Res.* 93: 237–248.

Haberly, l., and Bower, J. (1989) Olfactory cortex: model circuit for study of associative memory? *Trends in Neurosci.* 12:258–264.

Hakeem, A., McLaughlin, T., Sandoval, G., Jones, M., and Allman, J. (1994) Brain and life span in Primates, *Handbook of the Psychology of Aging.*

Hall, T., Miller, A., Corsellis, J, (1975) Variations in the human Purkinje cell population according to age and sex, *Neuropathol. Appl. Neurobiolog.* 1: 267–292.

Hoffman, M., Purba, J., and Swaab, D. (1993) Annual variations in the vasopressin neuron population of the human suprachiasmatic nucleus, *Neurosci.* 53:1103–1112.

Limonta, P., Maggi, R., Martini, L., and Piva, F., (1982) Role of the subcommissural organ in the control of gonadotrophin secretion in the female rat, *J. Endocrinol.*, 95: 207–213.

MacFarland, D. ed (1992) *Guinness Book of World Records*, Facts on File, New York.

Matano, S., Baron, G., Stephan, H., and Frahm, H. (1985) Volume comparisons in the cerebellar complex of Primates. II. Cerebellar nuclei. *Folia Primatol.* 44:182–203.

Mirmiran, M., Swaab, D., Kok, J., Hofman, M., Whitting, W., and Van Gool, W. (1992) Circadian rhythms and the suprachiasmatic nucleus in parental development, aging and Alzheimer's disease, *Prog. Brain Res.* 93: 151–163.

Moore, R. (1992) The organization of the human circadian timing system, *Prog. Brain Res.* 93:101–117.

Okawa, M., Hisikawa, Y., Hozumi, S., and Hori, H. (1991) Sleep-wake rhythm disorder and phototherapy in elderly patients with dementia, *Biol. Psychiatry* 29:161S–162S.

Quackenbush, L. and Pentney, R. (1990) Evidence for nonrandom regression of dendrites of Purkinje neurons during aging, *Neurobiol. Aging* 11:111–115.

Raz, N., Torres, I., Spencer, W., White, K., and Acker, J. (1992) Age-related regional differences in cerebellar vermis observed in vivo, *Arch. Neurol.* 49:412–416.

Rogers, J. (1988) The neurobiology of cerebellar senescence, *Ann N Y Acad Sci.*, 515:251–268.

Rogers, J., Zornetzer, S., and Bloom, F. (1981) Senescent pathology of cerebellum: Purkinje neurons and their parallel fiber afferents, *Neurobiol. Aging* 2:15–25.

Rogers, J., Zornetzer, S., Bloom F., and Mervis, R. (1984) Senescent microstructural changes in rat cerebellum, *Brain Res.* 292:23–32.

Ross, C. (1988) The intrinsic rate of natural increase and reproductive effort in primates, *J. Zool.* 214:199–219.

Sacher, G. (1975) Maturation and longevity in relation to cranial capacity in hominid evolution, In: Tuttle, R., ed., *Primate Functional Morphology and Evolution*, Mouton, The Hague, pp. 417–441.

Severs, W., Dundore, R., and Balaban, C. (1987) The subcommissural organ and Reissner's fibers: physiological regulation, In: Gross, P., ed., *Circumventricular Organs and Body Fluids*, Vol. II, CRC Press, Boca Raton, pp. 43–58.

Stephan, H., Baron, G., and Frahm, H. (1982) Comparison of brain structure volumes in insectivores and primates. II. Accessory olfactory bulb (AOB), *J. Hirnforsch.* 23:575–591.

Stephan, H., Frahm, H., and Baron, G., (1981) New and revised data on volumes of brain structures in insectivores and primates, *Folia Primatol.* 35:1–29.

Stephan, H., Frahm, H., and Baron, G. (1984) Comparison of brain structure volumes in insectivores and primates. IV. Non-cortical visual structures, *J. Hirnforsch.* 25:385–403.

Stephan, H., Frahm, H., and Baron, G. (1987) Comparison of brain structure volumes in insectivores and primates. VII. Amygdaloid components, *J. Hirnforsch.* 28:571–584.

Sturrock, R. (1989) A comparison of quantitative histological changes in different regions of the aging mouse cerebellum, *J. Hirnforsch.* 31:481–486.

Swaab, D., Hoffman, M., Lucassen, P., Purba, J., Raadsheer, F., and Van de Nes, J. (1993) Functional neuroanatomy and neuropathology of the human hypothalamus, *Anat. Embryol.* 187:317–330.

Takagishi, Y., and Yamamura, M. (1989) Purkinje cell abnormalities and synaptogensis in genetically jaundiced rats (Gunn rats), *Brain Res.* 492: 116–128.

Tideiksaar, R. and Fletcher, B. (1989) Keeping the elderly on their feet, *Iss. Sci. Technol.* 5:78–81.

Torvik, A., Lindboe, C., and Rogde, S. (1982) Brain lesions in alcoholics—a neuropathological study with clinical correlations, J. Neurolog. Sci. 56:233–248.

Torvik, A., and Torp, S. (1986) The prevalence of alcoholic cerebellar atrophy: a morphometric and histological study of an autopsy material. J. Neurolog. Sci. 75:43–51

Torvik, A., Torp S., and Lindboe, C. (1986) Atrophy of the cerebellar vermis in ageing: a morphometric and histologic study, *J. Neurol. Sci.* 76: 283–294.

Williams, R. and Herrup, K. (1988) The control of neuron number, *Ann. Rev. Neurosci.* 11:423–453.

Woodruff-Pak, D., Cronholm, J., and Sheffield, J. (1990) Purkinje cell number related to rate of classical conditioning, *Neuroreport* 1:165–168.

Woodruff-Pak, D., Steinmetz, J., and Thompson, R. (1988) Classical conditioning of rabbits 2 1/2 to 4 years old using mossy fiber stimulation as a CS, *Neurobiol Aging* 9(2):187–193.

Woodruff-Pak, D. and Thompson, R. (1988) Classical conditioning of the eyeblink response in the delay paradigm in adults ages 18–83 years, *Psychol Aging*: 3:219–229.

Zihlman, A., Morbeck, M., and Goodall, J. (1990) Skeletal biology and individual life history of Gombe chimpanzees, *J. Zool., Lond. 221*:37–61.

Zornetzer, S., Bloom, F., Mervis, R., and Rogers, J. (1981) Senescent changes in balance, coordination and cerebellar microanatomy, *Soc. Neurosci. Abstr.*7:690.

Index

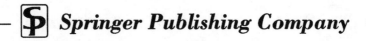
Springer Publishing Company

AGING AND MUSCULOSKELETAL DISORDERS
Concepts, Diagnosis, and Treatment

Horace M. Perry III, MD, John E. Morley, MD, BCh, and Rodney M. Coe, PhD, Editors

Describes the biomedical and environmental issues surrounding the loss of muscle and bone strength with age. Also covered are strategies for managing and decreasing risk of frailty, including exercise, nutritional, and hormonal interventions.

Partial Contents:

Part I. Epidemiology of Frailty in Older People. Epidemiology of Frailty: Scope of the Problem • Age-Related Changes in Bone: Longitudinal Study of Physical Performance and Frailty at Age 70 and Above

Part II. Age-Related Changes in Skeletal Muscle and Bone. Changes in Muscle Strength with Age • Cellular Basis of Aging in Skeletal Muscle • Changes in Bone Mass and Their Contribution to Fractures • Changes in Mineral and Bone Metabolism with Age • Osteoporosis in Post-Menopausal Women

Part III. Prediction and Prevention of Falls. Factors Contributing to Falls and Fractures • Epidemiology and Prevention of Falls in the Nursing Home • Adrenergic Receptors: Implications for Falls • Age-Related Changes in Balance: Rehabilitation Strategies

Part IV. Exercise, Nutrition, and Hormonal Interventions with the Frail Elderly. Effect of Exercise on Muscle Mass in the Elderly • Effect of Exercise on Bone Mass in the Elderly • Benefits of Exercise for the Elderly • Nutritional Intervention in the Frail Elderly • Meal-Associated Hypotension • Growth Hormone in Elderly Men

Part V. Rehabilitation of the Frail Elderly. An Update on The Diagnosis and Management of Musculoskeletal Disease in Older People • Nursing Rehabilitation of the Elderly Stroke Patient • Frailty and Physical Restraints • Posture Improvements in the Frail Elderly

1993   392pp   0-8261-7930-4   *hardcover*

536 Broadway, New York, NY 10012-3955 • (212) 431-4370 • Fax (212) 941-7842

THE BIOLOGY OF AGING

Richard L. Sprott, PhD,
Huber R. Warner, PhD, and
T. Franklin Williams, MD, Editors

Expert contributors provide valuable insights into the latest findings on biology and aging, including gene therapy, cancer biology, biology of Alzheimer's, stress and neuroendocrine change, as well as the ethics and future of aging research.

Contents:

1993   144pp   0-8261-8370-0   *hardcover*

536 Broadway, New York, NY 10012-3955 • (212) 431-4370 • Fax (212) 941-7842

WHO IS RESPONSIBLE FOR MY OLD AGE?

Robert N. Butler, MD, and
Kenzo Kiikuni, Editors

An insightful, international perspective on the "new gerontology." Emphasis is given to the notion that self-reliance among the aging cannot be achieved without active participation on the part of the entire community.

Contents:

1993   288pp   0-8261-8140-6   hardcover

536 Broadway, New York, NY 10012-3955 • (212) 431-4370 • Fax (212) 941-7842

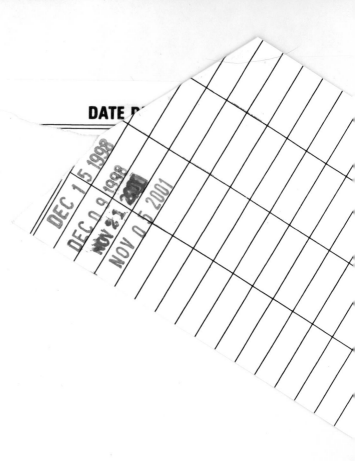